You Can Be...

Healthy & Fit After Fifty

*A Comprehensive Guide for Women & Men
Who Want to Achieve Health & Fitness*

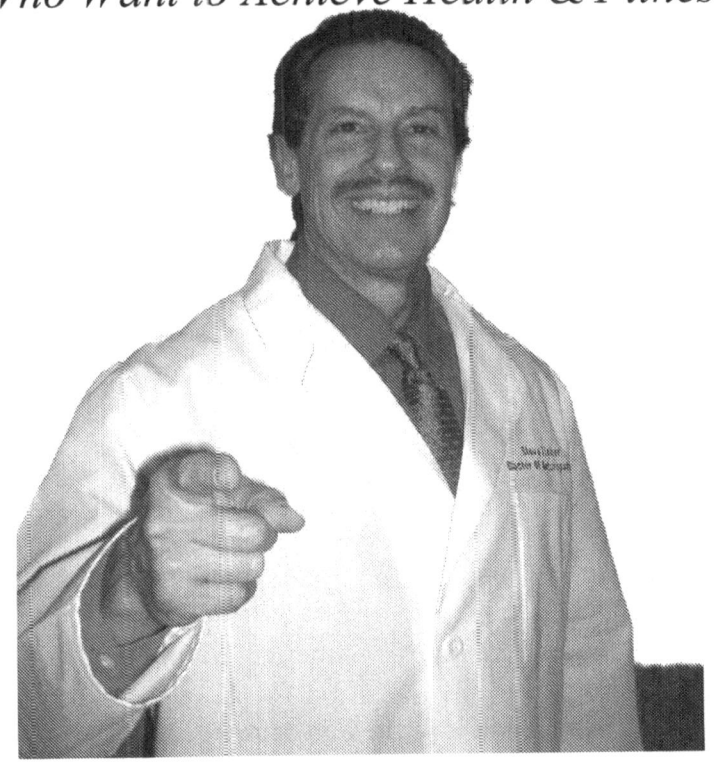

Steve Fisher, Doctor of Naturopathy

Healthy & Fit After Fifty

A Step by Step Comprehensive Guide for Women & Men
Who Want to Achieve Health and Fitness

Copyright © March 2007 U.S.
Copyright Registration Pending

Edited by Judy A. Hoofman: Texas2005@peoplepc.com

First published by AuthorHouse 10/10/07

ISBN: 978-1-4343-2390-3(soft)

Library of Congress Control Number: 2007905945

Printed in the United States of America, Bloomington, Indiana

This book is printed on acid-free paper.

Dedication

This book is dedicated to the memory of my beloved mother, who passed away while this book was in writing; to my son Gabriel, who preceded her; and to my father, who is alive and well. Heartfelt gratitude goes to my mother, who taught me the true meaning of unconditional love, and to my father, who taught me about commitment and hard work.

Special Thanks

Special thanks go out to each and every person who helped me with their personal bios and pictures. Without the input from these people and their modeling of all the exercises, this book would not have been the same. My appreciation goes to Cody and Marcia at Legends Gym for allowing me to take all of the exercise photos at their fine facility.

I want to add a special thanks to my spouse who has supported me in so many ways that it would take a whole chapter to list them all. The combination of the attributes gained from my parents and the help from my spouse made it possible for me to write this book, as I worked over fifty hours per week and maintained my health and fitness regime.

Table of Contents

Foreword

You cannot open a book without learning something.
Confucius

As a Naturopathic Doctor, I believe the human body was miraculously made. When placed in the right environment it can achieve amazing things. It has recently been reported that people should be living to one hundred and twenty years. Scientists have recently discovered that people will live this long when they are free of sickness and disease, or have the ability to overcome sickness and disease. The Bible states in Genesis 6:2 that man shall live one hundred and twenty years. Imagine that! The Bible and the scientific community coming to the same conclusion!

So if one hundred and twenty is the end of one's life, then fifty is not even the middle of a lifetime. For the sake of this book, I want you, the reader, to entertain me, and consider middle age to be fifty to one hundred, and one hundred and one to one hundred and twenty to be a senior citizen.

Now we must ask ourselves if living this long would even be pleasant. I believe it could be if we remain fit during the journey. If it were a simple task and everyone knew how to do it, or had the discipline to do it, we would certainly see a lot more people in their hundreds. I have talked to a lot of people about this subject, and it is quite interesting to note that people who smoke, drink excessively, or are generally unhealthy due to lifestyle habits seem to dislike the idea of living a long life, and those who are healthy and fit embrace the idea of a long life.

After pondering this for many years, I have come to the simple conclusion that people who are not healthy and fit just do not feel well most of the time, and a long life does not appeal to them for this reason. This is a problem that is fixable for those people living a life of misery due to lifestyles that are unhealthy! This book will give those people the tools to totally turn their lives around so that they

5

can feel so good that they would want to live a long life. Those who are already working on a healthy lifestyle will pick up pointers to further this endeavor.

Just recently it was reported by a local news station that a woman in DeKalb, Texas was one hundred and twenty-two years old. While this book was being written, this woman passed away during the month of October 2006. During the same month it was reported by the *Associated Press* that a man named Silas Simmons died. He was reported to be the oldest living man who had played professional baseball. Mr. Simmons was born the same year as Babe Ruth, in 1895, and was a pitcher and outfielder for a team in the Negro Leagues. He was one hundred and eleven years old when he died.

On Veteran's Day of 2006, there was a story in my local newspaper about twelve World War I vets who are still alive today. Their average age is one hundred and eight; with the oldest member being one hundred and fifteen. This gentleman now lives in Puerto Rico and credits his long life to his daily diet of boiled corn meal, cod, milk and a lifelong abstinence from alcohol. Another one of these men, who lives in West Virginia, still runs his three hundred and thirty acre farm and lives mostly on his own. Isn't this exciting to know that people are truly designed to live to one hundred and twenty years of life!

There was another gentleman on the news recently who is one hundred years old and still working at his western clothing business. His son, who is in upper seventies, was complaining that he couldn't retire yet because his father was still working. It made me laugh to hear about this son who is watching a living example of the way things should be. I must say that if one person can achieve this, so can you or I. We too can have children in their upper seventies complaining about not being able to retire because we are still working at something we enjoy doing, in our hundreds.

Another recent newspaper report told of a man, Waldo McBurney, who is one hundred and four years old and is still working on his honey farm. This gentleman works daily, and until a couple of years ago he competed in long distance running events. He didn't start long distance running until he was sixty five. Over the years he has accumulated ten gold medals in track and field at the Senior Olympics. When he was asked about retirement, he simply stated that retirement is not mentioned in The Bible. What an amazing story this is!

There is a man living in Georgia who is one hundred and five years old and still bowls regularly in two senior leagues, with an average of one hundred and six. He claims to be the world's oldest bowler. On Sundays he is driven to a church an hour and a half away and performs the task of ushering. He may also be the world's oldest usher! We hear about people living longer and remaining active all over the world. Once again I would say if he can do it, so can you or I.

In the November 2005 edition of *National Geographic* a study was discussed about the secrets of longevity. They observed the lives of advanced seniors living in Sardinia, Italy; Okinawa, Japan, and the Seventh Day Adventists living in California. A common thread that ran through all of their long lives was that all of them didn't smoke; they put their families first in their lives; all were active every day; and they all ate fruits, vegetables, and whole grains. The Okinawans keep lifelong friends, eat small portions of food, and find a strong purpose in their lives. The Sardinians drink red wine in moderation, share the work burden with their spouse, and eat foods that are high in omega-3 fatty acids. The Adventists eat nuts and beans, observe the Sabbath (which is Saturday for them), and have a strong faith in God. Many of these people are in their hundreds and still enjoying life performing daily activities that would seem difficult for people in their seventies.[1]

I have personally been on a health and fitness journey for many years now. My journey led me to the place I am at right now. It is a

---

[1] Buettner, D (2005, November), the Secrets of Long Life, National Geographic, 2 – 27.

place on the path, but I am far from arriving at the destination. I will endeavor to share my journey, along with the journey of others, who are also seeking the ultimate in health and fitness for themselves.

I challenge you, the reader, to join me on this journey and see where it will lead. I can personally guarantee you that it will add to the quality of your life and enhance the odds of living a longer life. You have nothing to lose, so why don't you place your feet on the path and begin your journey.

Introduction

You can't help getting older, but you don't have to get old.
George Burns

So now you're fifty. Where do you go from here? Is it going to be a downhill ride, or a road with peaks and valleys? Can I still look and feel good? Will I have the same health problems my parents had? Are you feeling uncertain about your future in regard to your health and fitness levels?

Well, you do not have to wonder about these questions any longer. The journey that you have begun will empower you with the knowledge to feel great and look even better. How do I know this is possible? Well, for one I have been over fifty for more than seven years now, and I've talked to many people who have achieved a high degree of health and fitness and are over fifty. I strongly believe that if one person can do something, then others can too!

The people I will mention in this book are people just like you. They are not professional models, ex-athletes, multi-millionaires, or movie stars. These people work and play the same as you and I. They've told me how they work on being healthy and fit, and I will pass that information along to you. Be aware that these people, like all people, are not perfect, and they too have flaws within themselves and their lifestyle. When these have been disclosed to me, I will pass that information along also. Many of these people have had medical problems in the past; some have even dealt with drug or alcohol addictions. I will reveal all of these issues also when they have been disclosed and I've been given permission to reveal.

Some of the questions that I asked these people are:
- What do you think is the most important factor in your present good health?
- What do you attribute to your above average level of fitness?
- How long do you think a person should live?

- At what age do you expect to see a decline in your health and fitness?
- Describe your exercise routine.
- Describe your eating and drinking patterns.
- Do you use any pharmaceutical drugs on a regular basis?
- Do you smoke or use any type of tobacco products?
- Do you drink alcoholic beverages? If so, how often and what type(s)?
- Do you take any nutritional supplements? If so, what types?
- How do you deal with stress?
- How would you rate your spiritual life?
- How do you keep your mind active?
- Discuss any health or fitness obstacles you've endured.

The people who were asked to participate are people that I personally know and believe to be healthy and fit. Many of them look years younger than their chronological age. Also keep in mind that people are not always one hundred percent truthful when answering questionnaires.

I've included pictures of these people that have not been touched up or changed in any manner. Look for the common threads that each of these people share and also look at the variety of their regimes. The small differences in their lifestyles could make a world of difference in yours.

Along with these testimonials I will give you the scientific reasons, in a language that you will understand, concerning the how and why fitness and health can be achieved and maintained after fifty.

There is a scientific term called "Expectation Theory." In short, this term tells us that in general the things we believe will happen usually do. If you expect to live a long and prosperous life, you probably will. On the other side of that coin, if you expect to live to seventy-five and have a decline in your health after fifty, you probably will. There is a proverb in the Bible that says, "As a man (or woman) thinks in his (or her) heart so he (or she) is." This was probably the

10

first time Expectation Theory was expressed in writing thousands of years ago.

Have you heard about the study done observing fleas? Flea trainers have observed a predictable and strange habit of fleas while training them. Fleas are trained by putting them in a cardboard box with a top on it. The fleas will jump up and hit the top of the cardboard box over and over again. As you watch them jump and hit the lid, something very interesting becomes obvious. The fleas continue to jump, but they are no longer jumping high enough to hit the top. Apparently, headache number two hundred and forty forces them to limit the height of their jump.

When you take off the lid, the fleas continue to jump, but they will not jump out of the box. They won't jump out because they think they can't jump out. Why? The reason is simple. They have conditioned themselves to jump just so high. Once they have conditioned themselves to jump just so high, that's all they can do!

Many times, people do the same thing. They restrict themselves and never reach their potential. Just like the fleas, they fail to jump higher, thinking they are doing all they can do.

As previously mentioned, a goal of this book is to empower you, the reader, with knowledge about health and fitness after the age of fifty, and another important goal is to change your expectation about how long and about the condition you will be in as you age. As we continue with our journey, I want you, the reader, to understand that there are numerous paths to any destination. What works for one person may not work for another. There are general guidelines that work for most people, but we must always be ready to adapt our health and fitness program to meet the individual need. These may include time, and, or money restraints. They may also include diverse physiological needs. Be flexible, try a variety of approaches, and you will be successful!

If you think you are beaten, you are. If you think you dare not, you don't! If you want to win, but think you can't, it's almost a cinch you won't. If you think you'll lose, you're lost; for out in the world we find Success begins with a fellow's will; it's all in the state of the mind. Life's battles don't always go to the stronger and faster man, but sooner or later the man who wins is the man who thinks he can.

Walter D. Wintle

The Components of Health & Fitness

Health

A journey of a thousand miles begins with a single step.
Confucius

What gives a person the right to claim he or she is healthy? In general it would be a person that is free of sickness and disease, and has an immune system with the ability to overcome sickness and disease. This person should also possess a sense of well-being. Does it mean that this person has never been sick, or that he will never become sick? No, it simply means that a person who is healthy can overcome illness and return to a state of being highly functional.

According to the *World Health Organization*, health is a state of complete physical, mental and social well-being and not merely the absence of disease or infirmity.

Health is metabolic efficiency. Sickness is metabolic inefficiency. Nobody is totally healthy or totally sick. Each of us is a unique combination of health and sickness. And each of us has a unique combination of abilities and disabilities, both emotional and physical.[2]

Health is a balance between your physical, mental and social well-being. Each of these three affects the others. If all three are balanced, then wellness is achieved and health is yours, but we must remember that any one of those aspects can negatively affect the other two.

---

[2] www.organicmd/whatishealth.html. 6/20/06.

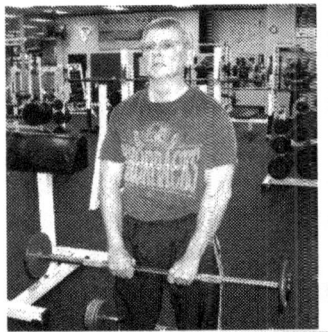

Wayland L. is a social worker who devotes himself to helping "at risk" juveniles find their way in society. He is sixty eight years young, and has been an inspiration to me for many years. I first met Wayland in a fitness center more than fifteen years ago, and he is truly a person who endeavors to be healthy and fit.

With the belief that diet and exercise are equally important, he works out three to four times per week at a fitness center, and limits white sugar, fried foods, red meat and foods that are high in sodium. He supplements his diet with a multi vitamin/mineral tablet, takes extra calcium/magnesium, and drinks a juice made from seaweed. Wayland also adds extra protein to his diet on a regular basis.

His stress management regime is to exercise, walk, and drive in the country. Wayland believes a person should live up to one hundred years, and he doesn't expect to see a decline in his fitness levels until he is in his mid seventies.

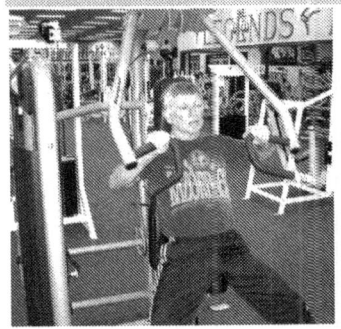

When asked about a health and fitness challenge in his life, he responded by telling me about a difficult divorce that he went through. This is just one more example of how it is impossible to separate the different aspects of our being. When we are emotionally upset it causes problems for us physically and spiritually.

Fitness

Doing the best at this moment puts you in the best place for the next moment.
Oprah Winfrey

What makes a person fit, and what are the markers for this? We can safely divide fitness into some basic categories. They are cardio-vascular (the health of the heart, lungs, veins, and arteries), plus strength (the ability for our skeletal system and muscles to exert force against an object), flexibility (the ability to stretch opposing muscle groups in a full range of motion), muscular endurance (the ability of a muscle to do sustained work), and the bodies composite (amount of muscle and fat it possesses).

Another definition of fitness, suited for the intellectual type, would be a state characterized by an ability to perform daily activities with vigor, and a demonstration of traits and capacities that are associated with low risk of premature development of the hypokinetic diseases.

Fitness can be defined in many different ways. To some people fitness might mean a slim waistline. To others it could be the ability to bench-press their body weight. And to others it might be a general feeling of wellness.

When you think of fitness, it's important to look at the big picture. It's not just about strength, endurance or fat content, but a combination of all these. You might be strong but have no endurance. You might have endurance but have little flexibility.

What you want to strive for is balance. Listed above are five key components important to a good definition of fitness. Investigate each one. Be totally honest with yourself! Consider areas where you are strong and the areas where you are weak. Strive to improve in all these areas, because the results will permeate your overall well-being.

Now that we have a clearer understanding of what health and fitness are, we can continue on our journey and begin to achieve this sought- after state of wellbeing that will enhance our lives richly.

Achieving Health

Nutritional Approach

*If we could give every individual the right amount of nourishment
and exercise, not too little and not too much, we would have found
the safest way to health.*

Hippocrates

The things we do today will either be to our benefit or detriment in
the future. In terms of our body's nutrition, we are often only as
good as our last meal.

Before I begin to tell you about the specifics of eating or drinking
for optimal health, I am going to explain some basic principles of
nutrition. I will endeavor to explain these in basic terms, but there
are some concepts that require the use of terminology that you may
not be accustomed to. So please bear with me, and I will guide you
through this important information. Remember, a portion of this
journey is gaining knowledge and insight, and the rest is the
utilization of this knowledge.

Nutrients are the food substances that an organism, or in our case the
human body, use for life functions. They can be divided into two
groups. One group supplies the building materials and fuel. This
group of nutrients includes proteins, carbohydrates, and fats (lipids),
and are they called macronutrients because they are used in large
amounts. The second group of nutrients is called micronutrients
because they are used in small quantities. These are the vitamins,
minerals, and other trace substances found in food, and are the tools
needed to make use of the building materials. A good example of
this would be if we were going to build a house we would purchase
the wood, nails, screws, pipes, cement, etc. and this would be
considered our macronutrients. Now we would need tools, such as
hammers, screwdrivers, drills, etc., to work with these materials to
make them into a house, and these tools would be our micronutrients.

Calories

It's hard for a day to go by without hearing about low calorie, restricted calories, reduced calories, or something about calories in relation to one's diet. So what exactly is a calorie? Calories are a unit of energy that is provided by foods. When averaged out, certain foods contain a set amount of calories. Carbohydrates and protein foods average approximately four calories per gram; while fats average nine calories per gram. A general rule is that if a person takes in more calories than they burn, they will gain weight; and if a person takes in fewer calories per day than they burn, they will lose weight. If the scale is balanced where the calories are equal to the amount burned, the person will maintain their current weight.

That seems to be fairly simple, but other factors can complicate the issue. First, it is quite hard to know exactly how many calories are actually in the foods we consume. It would require weighing everything we place in our mouth. Not a simple task to undertake! Next, we would have to know exactly how many calories are being used while performing the numerous day to day tasks that we do, and know the number of calories we burn while resting. This would take a monumental effort on one's part.

So, in my opinion, counting calories to maintain a healthy weight is not an option. What I have learned to do over the years is to eat more of certain foods, less of other foods, and eliminate some foods totally. This works well for me, and it doesn't take a rocket scientist to accomplish.

Proteins

Proteins provide essentially all the structural elements, the transport systems, and the control mechanisms of the human body. When necessary they can be metabolized to provide heat and energy required for life functions, but protein is not the most efficient fuel. Ideally carbohydrates and fats better accomplish energy production.

Proteins are so important to the human body that they are required to some degree by every structure or function.

The building blocks of protein are called amino acids. There are more than forty naturally occurring amino acids. Of all the amino acids only nine are considered essential. These proteins are considered essential because the human body cannot produce or convert other amino acids to these. When a protein food has all the essential amino acids it is called a complete protein. Animal proteins are generally of this type, with the exception of gelatin. When a food does not possess all of the essential amino acids it is considered an incomplete protein, which is generally found in plant proteins, with the exception of soybeans. Thus it becomes important to eat the right plant proteins in combination in order to get a complete protein. Vegetarians must be careful to learn how to accomplish this, or they will suffer from protein deficiencies.

Protein foods are rated by their digestibility and biological value. Whole eggs are usually at the top of most of these charts, with your meat and other dairy products following. Vegetable protein sources are at the end of these charts. The importance of dietary protein cannot be overstated. It is essential for maintaining and repairing muscle tissue and provides the ingredients to make enzymes, hormones, and many other biochemicals that are so important to good health and well-being.

Carbohydrates

In actuality there are no carbohydrates that are essential for humans, yet carbohydrate foods are very important vehicles for countless essential micronutrients. Fruits and vegetables are a major source of fiber, minerals, and vitamins, especially Vitamin A, C, and E. They are also the only sources of important phytochemicals such as carotenoids and bioflavonoids. Glucose derived from carbohydrates serves as an important source of energy, and as the blood component that helps the body maintain homeostasis (the internal stability of the

19

body). A minimum of twenty percent of a diet should be unrefined carbohydrates.[3]

For those of you who are on the extremely low carbohydrate diets I want you to understand the importance of unrefined carbohydrates. Many important nutrients and necessary fiber is brought into our bodies via unrefined carbohydrates. Some of these nutrients are quite difficult to receive without the addition of unrefined carbohydrates in our daily diets. This will be discussed in greater detail later on in this book.

Unfortunately, most Americans take in carbohydrates in the form of refined, meaning they have been highly processed. People with high cholesterol levels have to understand that most cholesterol found in the blood is manufactured by their own body's biochemistry. The major cause of cholesterol in the blood is refined carbohydrates, not saturated fat.

White sugar and white flour are two of the most dangerous villains in our diets today, and they should be avoided at all costs. They are the culprits in heart disease, type II diabetes, and countless other diseases and even emotional disorders. As a part of our journey I want you to consider these villains as the pop-up bad guys in a video game that are trying to take you out!

If you were to simply eliminate all forms of white sugar and white flour from your diet, you would be taking huge steps in your journey, and would feel and look better in a very short period of time. So remember to avoid, or blast these villains out of your path while you travel on your journey.

Approximately three and a half years ago I eliminated white sugar, white flour and white rice from my diet. I did this in an attempt to

---

[3] Ottoboni, Alice & Ottobon., Fred, (2002) The Modern Nutritional Diseases and how to prevent them, Vincente Books Inc.

be healthier, but to my surprise I began to lose weight without adjusting anything else in my diet or exercise program. In fact, I lost approximately fifteen pounds in six months and then it leveled off to where I am today. Think about that for a moment. You can eat the same amount of food, but change this simple feature and lose weight. Simply replace the refined carbohydrates with unrefined carbohydrates. You will be given more information about this as we move forward in our journey.

Fats

Fat is a word we've all come to loathe. It conjures up visions of grease, overweight people, and something that will cause us to become unhealthy. In my opinion fat has been given a bad rap. For years we've been told to avoid this nasty substance, yet at the same time we all know how good it makes things taste. So what should the average person do about fat in his or her diet?

While fat is generally considered to be a negative thing, it is an essential part of the diet. There are three different types of fat: saturated, unsaturated, and trans-fatty acids. Saturated fat, which is found in foods such as meat, poultry, lard, palm oil, coconut oil, and whole milk, should be consumed in small quantities. It is recommended that saturated fat make up no more than 10% of the diet, and I would agree with this general recommendation. To accomplish this, eat lean cuts of meat, avoid deep fried foods, and limit your dairy products.

In reading most standard health literature you will find that saturated fat has become synonymous with the term, "cholesterol buildup." When hearing this information I want to caution the reader into another line of thinking about cholesterol. Your liver produces cholesterol when you take in refined carbohydrates such as white sugar and white flour. This cholesterol has been proven to enter your bloodstream, and in my opinion is the culprit for the cholesterol that blocks your arteries and causes heart disease. Yes, I agree that we must limit saturated fat in our diet, but it is probably of greater importance to limit or totally eliminate these refined carbohydrates as well.

Unsaturated fat is found in oils such as olive oil, vegetable oil, and sunflower oil. This form of fat should account for about approximately 20 % of the diet, with the majority coming from monosaturated fats found in olive oil, avocados, canola and raw unsalted nuts and seeds.

The last type of fat is trans-fatty acid, which is formed when hydrogen is combined with unsaturated fat to make it a solid. Trans-fats should be avoided in all foods. They are manmade through a chemical process called hydrogenation that allows foods to look better, spread easier, resist high temperatures, remain non-smoking when heated, and have a longer shelf life. These types of fats interfere with biochemical processes, such as the metabolism of essential fatty acids, decrease good cholesterol (HDL), increase harmful cholesterol (LDL), and raise blood glucose levels. Trans-fats have been implicated in the causation of heart disease and cancer.

Foods such as peanut butter and margarine are two examples of this process called hydrogenation that produces trans-fats as a by-product. If you buy a bottle of organic peanut butter, you will notice the peanut oil is on the top portion of the jar. This is because it has not been chemically altered. Just recently you might have noticed that foods now tell you how many trans-fats they contain. This is really helpful in an attempt to avoid these products. They should also be treated as villains out to get you. Stay clear of these guys!

Do not be afraid to include fats in your diet, but try to include the healthier fats mentioned, and once again I want to say that it is extremely important to stay away from all trans-fat in your diet.

Water

After oxygen, water is the most important nutrient for the body. The human body is composed of approximately sixty-seven percent water. We can go without food for thirty to forty days, but without water our lives would end in three to five days.

It is almost impossible to drink too much water. The majority of people are chronically dehydrated, and a lack of water is the number one cause of daytime fatigue. Even a mild case of dehydration can slow a person's metabolism down by three percent, and a two percent drop in body water can cause fuzzy short term memory trouble with basic math and make it difficult to focus on a computer screen, or on printed material. With this is mind employers would be wise to make good quality water available for all their employees. It should pay for itself in productivity.

Research has indicated that eight to ten glasses of water per day could significantly reduce arthritis, back, and joint pain for almost eighty percent of sufferers. Water can be a fantastic aid to people trying to reduce their caloric intake. In a University of Washington study it was shown that just one glass of water stopped midnight hunger pangs for almost one hundred percent of dieters studied.

Drinking a glass of water thirty minutes before a meal can assist a dieter by eliminating those strong feelings of hunger. I do want to caution everyone to watch their fluid intake during meals because this practice will dilute your digestive enzymes. So try to consume the majority of water before meals or an hour after meals.

Drinking five glasses of water daily decreases the risk of breast cancer by seventy-nine percent, and a person is fifty percent less likely to develop bladder cancer. Quality water is beneficial for virtually all disorders known to mankind. If you have a desire to learn even more about the wonders of water you should read, *Your Body's Many Cries for Water*, by Dr. Batmanghelidj.

Not all water is as beneficial as other water sources. Almost all tap water is unfit to drink. It contains numerous harmful chemicals and impurities. You should drink filtered water when possible. There are many types of filtration systems being used. A reverse osmosis system with a carbon filter is one of the better filtration systems available, but I realize that cost does matter to most of us. I would recommend you use the best one you can afford without having to sell your firstborn child (although that may appeal to some of you).

I generally recommend sixty-four to eighty ounces of water per day, depending on a person's size. I have personally seen remarkable results from the increase of pure water consumed on a daily basis. You cannot be healthy without drinking the right amount of water on a daily basis!

Fiber

Let's take a brief look at fiber. Dietary fiber can help a person look and feel better. A recent study published in the Journal of the *American Dietetic Association* found that the main difference between "normal weight" adults and their overweight counterparts was the amount of fiber they consumed. Fiber swells in your belly and fills you up. It digests slowly and adds bulk (the indigestible part) to the diet. It also helps to stabilize blood sugar levels, which helps to prevent the peaks and valleys that cause a person to want to attack anything in the fridge, and it helps to reduce the risk of Type II Diabetes.

Fiber is also extremely important for gastrointestinal health, especially for the fifty plus group. It also contains a healthy dose of disease fighting antioxidants.[4] Remember, the main benefit of fiber is to promote easy elimination and help the digestive system to function optimally. In most cases constipation comes about because there are insufficient amounts of fiber and fluid in the diet.

---

[4] http://diets.aol.com/newsandtrends/highfiber, Fiber Up to slim Down, Patural, Amy, 6/27/06.

Fiber is also helpful in removing certain toxic metals. There are seven classifications of fiber: bran, cellulose, gum, hemicelluose, lignin, mucilages, and pectin. It is advisable to rotate your fiber sources when possible. A general rule is to start with small sources and gradually increase your intake until your stools are a good consistency.

Plant foods are the only dietary source of fiber. It is mainly cellulose, the structural part of a plant. You will find it in whole grains, fruits and vegetables. Try to include whole grain cereals and flours, brown rice, agar, all types of bran, fresh fruits, dried prunes, nuts, seeds (especially flaxseeds), beans, lentils, peas, and fresh raw vegetables.

Fiber that is soluble in water will help to soften stools, and the insoluble fiber passes through the intestine largely unchanged and adds bulk to the stool (which stimulates bowel contractions).

If you decide to use supplemental fiber it should always be taken separately from other medications or supplements because it can lessen their strength and effectiveness.

One of the ways you can tell when a person has reached middle age (remember that is fifty to one hundred years young) is when they can talk about bowel movements without being embarrassed, or at times with pride.

Glycemic Index

You have probably heard the term, "Glycemic index" used in reference to some diets that are popular. The glycemic index is a measure of the rate at which glucose from any given food enters the blood. Glucose is taken as the standard measurement and is assigned the number one hundred. Other foods are then compared to glucose and also assigned a number. Fructose, which is fruit sugar, is a twenty on the glycemic index. The general concept here is that the lower the glycemic index rating of the foods you ingest, the lower your blood glucose levels will be. This is especially important to people with Type I Diabetes, or Type II Diabetes.

Products that are high in sugars, refined flour, or starchy vegetables have high glycemic index numbers and should be avoided, or taken in moderation. Proteins and fats have a glycemic index number of zero. Generally foods that are high on the glycemic index also have a lot of calories. These foods tend not to satisfy hunger. People who have weight problems will be interested to know that nutritional research confirms this belief and even gives some explanation. One specific study found that high glycemic carbohydrates might promote hunger.[5] Another study postulates that the rapid absorption of glucose from high glycemic foods induces a sequence of hormonal and metabolic changes that promote excessive food intake.[6]

Here is a little guide to help you stay on the lower half of the glycemic index:

- Do not eat table sugar (sucrose) in any form.
- Eliminate nearly all white potatoes. Instead, choose a small sweet potato or a small portion of red-skinned potatoes.
- Never eat white bread. Delicious 100% whole grain breads are now widely available. Buy thinly sliced bread when possible and limit yourself to one portion.
- When buying pasta, look for whole grain. Remember, more fiber means a lower GI, and keep your portions to ½ cup until you see how your body reacts.
- Corn should be avoided.
- Avoid white rice. Whole grain brown rice is a better choice.
- Limit yourself to long cooking non-instant oatmeal rather the quick cooking varieties, and sweeten it with a low GI fruit.

---

[5] Roberts, S.B. High glycemic index foods, hunger, and obesity: is there a connection? *Nutrition Reviews. 2000; 58 (6): 163-9.*
[6] Ludwig, D.S.., et al. High glycemic index foods. Overeating, Obesity. and *Pediatrics.* 1999; 103(3): E26.

- Avoid tropical fruits like pineapple and watermelon. Instead, choose more temperate fruits like pears, apples, cherries and peaches.
- Keep your portions of carbohydrates small. Try to stay around ½ cup. Consuming a higher portion of protein and green or leafy vegetables can help you resist the temptation to overindulge in carbohydrates.
- Cook with healthy fats. These fats slow down the absorption of carbohydrates and often speed your metabolism. Healthy fats include mono-unsaturated like olive oil and peanut oil. Even real butter, a good source of CLA, is now considered a healthy fat.
- Nuts make a great low glycemic snack and deliver healthy monounsaturated to your body. Add some macadamia nuts, peanuts and walnuts to your diet.
- Adding acid to your food helps to lower the GI of the food. Use lemon juice and apple cider vinegar when you prepare foods and choose salad dressings that are apple cider vinegar and oil based.
- When you are reading labels, choose the products higher in dietary fiber for a lower GI.

One of the most rewarding aspects of choosing foods based on the glycemic index is that you will begin to realize that you do not feel as hungry. The carbohydrate cravings will lessen. Your body will be getting the nutrition it needs rather than empty calories. Promoting a healthy lifestyle is a powerful prevention for a number of illnesses.

Recommendations

Now you ask which foods should you eat and which ones should you avoid. At fifty years young, do you have to modify your eating habits? The answer to this is definitely "yes." As we age our metabolism gets slower and we require fewer calories; thus, we must make adjustments to our diet. Years ago I remember eating almost anything and still not getting fat, but those days are gone! As a child my mother gave me all types of calorie laden food (which I enjoyed very much) in an endeavor to help me gain weight. As I aged I noticed that there was a period of time when this was no longer necessary, approximately twenty-five for me, and then came the time that I had to be careful not to eat the wrong foods too often or I would pay for it in the form of a larger waistline. This seemed to start around the age of forty-five.

Some people are blessed in that they can eat all types of food and never gain unwanted fat around the midsection. In my opinion this is a two edged sword. Even though a person doesn't get fat when eating the junk foods, he or she can still be setting themselves up for sickness and disease.

We can do things to keep our system running efficiently, but even when we do all the things necessary to accomplish this, we will still have a slower metabolism than we did twenty years ago. So we must adjust our eating habits accordingly.

Ideally we should consume approximately fifty percent (sixty percent if we are dealing with sickness or disease) of our diet in the form of vegetables and fruits. That leaves fifty percent for protein foods, healthy fats, and our unrefined carbohydrates (other than the vegetables and fruits). I'll give you more details on this as we go on. Let's talk about the fruit and vegetable intake for a moment. Of that fifty percent, approximately thirty-five percent should be in the form of vegetables. About half of those should be raw and the rest steamed or cooked. If possible eat organic produce because they are produced without the use of pesticides, herbicides, and synthetic fertilizers that may cause harm in the form of sickness and disease to your body. A simple method to ensure variety to your produce is to eat a variety of colored produce. That is green, yellow, orange, red, purple, etc. On a regular basis include broccoli, cauliflower, onions, garlic, tomatoes, peppers, spinach, squash, beans, and others that you will find listed as natural sources of vitamins and minerals. These are all super foods that will help us to achieve the state of wellness that we are seeking.

Eat a variety of fruits on a regular basis also. Be sure to include various berries, apples, oranges, bananas (in moderation due to the fact that they are high on the glycemic index), melons, and others that you will find listed as natural sources of vitamins and minerals. Most fruits should be eaten in the raw state, but they can be cooked to make tasty desserts or additions to your cereal.

To simplify this eating arrangement, your plate should consist of half of its content in the form of vegetables and fruits. The remaining half of your plate should consist of healthy protein, healthy fats, and other unrefined carbohydrates. The majority of this part of your plate will be the protein portion. Your protein should come from what is known as "free range animals." A free range animal is one that has been allowed to roam and graze a given area for their food sources, and they have not been given antibiotics or growth hormones. Most of these products are more costly than the regular animal products out there, but they are well worth it if it is feasible within your budget.

Chicken, turkey, beef (in moderation), bison, wild animals such as deer, rabbit, etc., wild cold water fish, soy products, dairy products (in moderation), beans, legumes, and eggs should be the mainstay for your protein. The reader must understand that most foods are a combination of proteins, fats, and at times carbohydrates. With that in mind I have listed foods that are primarily from the category we are discussing.

The other twenty percent of your diet should come from healthy fats, and unrefined carbohydrates. Healthy fats are in walnuts, almonds, peanuts, cashews, macadamia nuts, pumpkin seeds, avocados, fish oil, flaxseed oil, olive oil, coconut oil, canola oil, etc.... You should eat nuts or seeds that are raw or dry roasted without added salt.

Unrefined carbohydrates are an important source of fiber. These can be found in fresh fruits, dried fruits, vegetables, whole grains such as brown rice, 100% whole wheat in bread or pasta, sprouted grains, and whole grain cereals such as oats. Other types of whole grains are barley, buckwheat, amaranth, bulgar, corn, kamut, quinoa, rye, spelt, teff, and wild rice.

The fruits and vegetables do not count in this portion of the percentage because we have already counted them in the first fifty percent group. So, we include the other unrefined carbohydrates and healthy fats as the other twenty percent of the diet.

It is generally a good idea to have some protein with any carbohydrates ingested. This ensures a good mix of hormones that will be produced (i.e. insulin is produced from carbohydrates ingested, and glucagon is produced when proteins are ingested). Insulin and glucagon are secreted by cells in the pancreas and then brought in the bloodstream to all the cells of the body where they control cellular metabolism through regulation of various biochemical processes. This is an oversimplification of the process, but enough to give the reader some understanding of the reason to try balance the various types of food to be ingested.

Try not to complicate your nutritional plan. I realize this is easier said than done because of all the information a person must sort through and learn to incorporate to make a healthy and practical nutritional regime. The percentages given are approximations to give you an idea of what you should be shooting for. You must also remember that we are trying to eat five to six small meals per day, so these foods will be divided among these meals.

If you simply avoid the harmful foods and beverages discussed later in this book, and use the basic principles outlined throughout your reading, you should do all right. Refer to the chapter on things to avoid to remain healthy for a detailed listing of harmful foods. Remember this is a journey, not a destination. Your diet will evolve over time and you can progressively improve upon it.

Anyone who stops learning is old, whether at twenty or eighty.
Anyone who keeps learning stays young. The greatest thing in life is
to keep your mind young.
Henry Ford

My Personal Nutritional Regime

I always start my day with a glass of filtered water before eating anything. This can serve you in a number of positive ways. It will get your digestive juices flowing, and it will help to keep your appetite suppressed to some degree, and it will help to hydrate your body after a good night's sleep.

My breakfast consists of non-instant organic oatmeal with organic blueberries, organic raisins, organic cinnamon, organic milk, and a scoop of whey protein. I alternate this with an organic dry cereal, added organic berries, organic raisins, and a scoop of whey protein. I rarely deviate from these two breakfasts. I know I was redundant in mentioning organic products numerous times, but I feel it is important to use products that are free of insecticides, pesticides, hormones, antibiotics, and artificial fertilizers whenever it is feasible. For the rest of this book I will not mention whether or not the foods I use are organic or not. That will be up to the reader's discretion.

I do understand that many of our readers cannot afford to purchase these products, so by all means just use whatever you can afford. As long as you adhere to the basic nutritional guidelines outlined, you will benefit.

My snacks are eaten between my breakfast and lunch and between my lunch and supper. For a snack I usually have raw nuts (almonds, walnuts, cashews, pumpkin seeds, etc.) with a fruit. I may deviate from this according to availability and ability to access (when away from my home or workplace) various snack items.

My lunch and supper varies quite a bit, but I will give you some idea of what I generally eat. I try to have one protein dish, which is about one third of the meal, and an assortment of vegetables, either cooked or raw. If I eat bread it will be a sprouted variety such as Ezekiel Bread. Instead of using margarine or butter (which I use occasionally) on bread, I may put some olive oil on it. I also do this with whole grain crackers.

Some of my favorite dishes are stir fry with bean sprouts, broccoli, cauliflower, carrots, tuna, cheese, Bragg's Liquid Aminos (tastes just like soy sauce), grated peppers, and canola oil. Canola oil holds up better than olive oil when heated, and is quite reasonable in price. Other dishes include omelets made with free range eggs, buffalo dogs (hot dogs made with bison meat), chicken, and assorted vegetables, whole grain pasta, with basil and parmesan cheese, brown rice, wild salmon and vegetables; and occasionally I will eat a sweet potato.

During the day I try to ingest approximately seventy to eighty ounces of pure filtered water. I drink this throughout the day. After a weight bearing workout, I usually drink a glass of cow, or soy milk with whey protein added to it. I will discuss this further when we talk about supplementation.

For a treat I enjoy fat free, no sugar added TCBY ice cream, chocolate soymilk, spoonfuls of natural peanut or cashew butter mixed with honey, and popcorn.

Supplementation

Supplementation is an extremely controversial issue. You will find professionals telling you that you must use mega doses of certain nutrients to achieve wellness, and then on the other side of this spectrum, you will find other professionals saying that a healthy person with an adequate diet should not need any additional supplements. You've probably heard about miracle juices and herbs that can cure everything and anything. This leaves the average person scratching his or her head and wondering if anyone really knows the truth.

Well, the truth lies within you. Each and every person has a different physiological makeup and we must experiment, within certain guidelines, to figure out which things work best for us. The right amount of one nutrient for one person may be an overdose for another person. Without a shadow of doubt I believe the best nutrients are found in our foods, and we should strive to get our nutrients from our diets!

If we lived in an ideal world with endless cash flow, we could eat all of our nutrients in the form of organic fruits, organic vegetables, free-range produce and meats, organic seeds and nuts, etc. The list could go on and on. I, personally, have not achieved that standard of living as of the writing of this book. Thus I will approach this from the perspective of an average person with an average income.

Everyone should take a whole food multiple vitamin and mineral supplement on a daily basis. Even if you eat well, this serves as an insurance policy. In other words, it will ensure that you are getting the nutrients you need. Something a person should be aware of is the percent of absorption of the supplements we take. Most supplements we take orally are going to give us an absorption rate of approximately twenty-five percent. This means that we are not absorbing seventy-five percent of the supplement. When we take something sublingually (that is when you place the supplement under your tongue) the absorption rate goes up into the low thirty-percentile area. When taken in an intramuscular shot we absorb about seventy percent, and if the shot is intravenous then the absorption rate is approximately one hundred percent. I do not recommend getting your nutrients using a needle unless you are under the care of a physician that deems it necessary, because there are risk factors in doing so.

Find a whole food multi-vitamin/mineral that helps you to feel better than when you are not taking the supplemental vitamin/mineral. Give a supplement a good three to four weeks to test it out. Ask yourself questions like "Do I have more energy now?" "Is my strength increasing?" "Am I sleeping better?" and "Are the problems subsiding that prompted me to take the supplement in the first place?"

Antioxidants are very important for people over fifty. An anti-oxidant is a substance that protects our cells from free radical damage. A free radical cell is one that is missing an electron and searches for one to steal from another cell. This causes cell mutation and can lead to sickness and disease.

At this point I am going to tell you about most of the antioxidants, vitamins, minerals, herbs, and other healthy supplements. You, the reader, will have to evaluate the ones that you think will help you and then experiment with your different choices to see what makes the most positive effects in your life.

Always remember to ask yourself certain questions when someone is telling you about any nutritional product. These questions are: Is this person going to benefit financially from my using this product? Is the research on this product done by an independent source, not the company that is selling the product? Can I afford to use this product on a regular basis? Can I get the same product of equal quality cheaper from another source? Is there anything in this product that may interact in a negative fashion with any pharmaceutical drugs that I am taking? Be aware that most medical doctors are not familiar with natural supplemental products and will generally tell their patients to stay away from them because they do not possess the knowledge to administer them safely.

In this day and age it seems as though it is hard to find a person who is trustworthy, but if a person does not have anything to gain financially from your purchase and if they are truly interested in your health and well-being, they will give you the best advice they

34

are capable of giving. A good person to consult with would be a naturopathic doctor that is not representing any company or product. This person will only gain something if you do well.

I had the thought about creating a health care system where you only paid when you were free of sickness and disease. Can you imagine how hard the practitioners would be trying to get you well and to help you stay well? They wouldn't be able to stay in business long if all of their patients were ill and never paying their premiums due to sickness. Well, enough daydreaming; let's move forward in our journey and learn about the supplements that can assist us in our endeavor to be healthy and fit.

Listed below are some of the vitamins, minerals, antioxidants, amino acids, herbs, and other nutrients that I feel are important for a person over fifty, and I'll give you a brief synopsis about each of them. Once again, I want to remind you that the best sources of nutrients are from the original source, being food; thus you will find the natural sources for each of these supplements. Look at these natural sources and try to include as many of these as possible in your daily diet.

Vitamins

Vitamins function mainly as coenzymes (that is, they work in conjunction with enzymes) to perform a variety of metabolic reactions and biochemical mechanisms within our numerous bodily systems. Most vitamins cannot be manufactured by the body, with the exception of some B vitamins or when beta-carotene is converted to Vitamin A.

Most vitamin supplements are better absorbed when taken with food, but once again I will reiterate that the best way to get your nutrition is by eating a nutritious diet on a regular daily basis.

There are basically two types of vitamins: water-soluble vitamins (Vitamin C and the B vitamins), and fat-soluble vitamins (vitamins A, D, E, and K). Let's take a look at these vitamins and find out exactly what they do for us.

Vitamin A: Helps to prevent night blindness and other eye problems, as well as some skin disorders, such as acne. It enhances the immune system and may help to heal gastrointestinal ulcers, and is needed for maintenance and repair of epithelial tissue, of which the skin and mucous membranes are composed. It is important in the formation of bones and teeth, aids in fat storage, and protects against colds, flu, and other infections of the kidneys, bladder, lungs, and mucous membranes. It also acts as an antioxicant, helping to protect the cells against cancer and other diseases. Applied topically it aids in reducing wrinkles (used in Retin-A and Renova).

Sources of this vitamin are found in animal livers, fish liver oils, green and yellow vegetables and fruits. An abundant source is found in apricots, beet greens, broccoli, cantaloupe, carrots, collards, dandelion greens, dulse, fish liver and fish liver oil, garlic, kale, mustard greens, papayas, peaches, pumpkin, red peppers, spinach, spirulina, sweet potatoes, Swiss chard, turnip greens, watercress, and yellow squash.[7]

Always be cautious to not exceed the recommended dosage on labels or the one given by your health practitioner when supplementing Vitamin A.

Q: What's the difference between a general practitioner and a specialist?
A: One treats what you have; the other thinks you have what he treats.

Vitamin B1 (Thiamine): enhances circulation and assists in blood formation, carbohydrate metabolism, and the production of

---

[7] Phyllis A. Balch, CNC & James F. Balch, MD (2000) Prescription for Nutritional Healing, Avery Books, 13 - 14.

hydrochloric acid, which is important for proper digestion. This vitamin also optimizes cognitive activity and brain function. It also acts as an antioxidant, protecting the body from the degenerative effects of aging, alcohol consumption, and smoking.

The richest food sources of this vitamin are brown rice, egg yolks, fish, legumes, peanuts, liver, peas, pork, poultry, rice bran, wheat germ, and whole grains. [8]

Vitamin B2 (Riboflavin): is necessary for red blood formation, antibody production, cell respiration, and growth. It helps to alleviate eye fatigue and is important in the prevention and treatment of cataracts. It aids in the metabolism of carbohydrates, fats and protein. Together with Vitamin A, it maintains and improves the mucous membranes in the digestive tract. Vitamin B2 also facilitates the use of oxygen by the tissues of the skin, nails, and hair; eliminates dandruff, and helps the absorption of iron, and Vitamin B6.

High levels of B2 are found in cheese, egg yolks, fish legumes, meat, milk, poultry, spinach, whole grains, and yogurt. Oral contraceptives and strenuous exercise increase the need for this vitamin.

Vitamin B3 (Niacin, Nicotinic Acid, and Niacinamide): is needed for proper circulation and healthy skin. It aids in the functioning of the nervous system; in the metabolism of carbohydrates, fats, and proteins; and in the production of hydrochloric acid. It is also involved in the normal secretion of bile and stomach fluids, and in the synthesis of sex hormones. Niacin lowers cholesterol and improves circulation.

Niacin and Niacinamide are found in beef liver, brewer's yeast, broccoli, carrots, cheese, corn flour, dandelion greens, dates, eggs, fish, milk, peanuts, pork, potatoes, tomatoes, wheat germ, and whole-wheat products.

---

[8] Ibid, 16

People who are pregnant or who suffer from diabetes, glaucoma, gout, liver disease, or peptic ulcers should use niacin with caution.

Doctor: The tests show that your cancer is advanced and you have only six months to live!

Patient: But, doc, I can't pay all of my medical bills in six months!

Doctor: In that case, you have twelve months to live.

Vitamin B5 (Pantothenic Acid): is also known as the anti-stress vitamin. It plays a role in the production of the adrenal hormones and the formation of antibodies, aids in vitamin utilization, and helps to convert fats, carbohydrates, and proteins into energy. It is required by all cells in the body and is concentrated in the organs. Vitamin B5 is also involved in the production of neurotransmitters.

Sources of this vitamin are beef, brewer's yeast eggs, fresh vegetables, kidney, legumes, liver, mushrooms, nuts, pork, royal jelly, saltwater fish, torula yeast, whole rye flour, and wheat flour.[9]

Vitamin B6 (Pyridoxine): is involved in more bodily functions than almost any other single nutrient. It affects both physical and mental health. It is involved in the production of hydrochloric acid, and is necessary for the absorption of fats and protein. It helps to maintain the mineral balance of sodium and potassium; promotes red blood cell formation; is required by the nervous system, and is needed for normal brain function. The list goes on further, but these are the main functions the reader should know about.

Almost all foods contain some B6, but the following foods have the highest amounts: brewer's yeast, carrots, chicken, eggs, fish, meat, peas, spinach, sunflower seeds, walnuts, and wheat germ.

Antidepressants, estrogen therapy, and oral contraceptives may increase the need for this vitamin. Also note that diuretics and

---

[9] Ibid, 17

cortisone drugs block the absorption of Vitamin B6. Prolonged use of high doses (over 1,000 mg. per day of B6) can be toxic and may result in nerve damage and loss of concentration.

Vitamin B12 (Cyanobalamin): is needed to prevent anemia. It aids folic acid in regulating the formation of red blood cells, and helps in the utilization of iron. It is required for proper digestion, absorption of foods, the synthesis of protein, and the metabolism of carbohydrates and fats. It also aids in cell formation and cellular longevity; prevents nerve damage, maintains fertility, and promotes normal growth and development.

The largest amounts of B12 are found in brewer's yeast, clams, eggs, herring, kidney, liver, mackerel, milk and dairy products, and seafood. It is not found in many vegetables, with sea vegetables being the main exception.

Anti-gout medications, anticoagulant drugs, and potassium supplements may block absorption of Vitamin B12. [10]

Folate (Folacin, Folic Acid, or PGA): is considered a brain food, and is needed for energy production and the formation of red blood cells. It also strengthens the immune system by aiding in the formation of white blood cells. It is important for healthy cell division and replication, and is involved in protein metabolism. This nutrient may also help in the treatment of depression and anxiety.

Sources of Folate are asparagus, barley, beef, bran, brewer's yeast, brown rice, cheese, chicken, dates, green leafy vegetables, lamb, legumes, lentils, liver, milk, mushrooms, oranges, split peas, pork, root vegetables, salmon, tuna, wheat germ, whole grains, and whole wheat.

Oral contraceptives may increase the need for folate.

---

[10] Ibid, 18

Inositol: is vital for hair growth; has a calming effect, and helps to reduce cholesterol. There is some research that indicates that high doses of inositol may help in the treatment of depression, obsessive-compulsive disorder, and anxiety disorders without the side effects of prescription drugs.

Sources of inositol are brewer's yeast, fruits, lecithin, legumes, meats, milk, unrefined molasses, raisins, vegetables, and whole grains. Consumption of a large amount of caffeine may cause a shortage of inositol in the body.[11]

Vitamin C: is an antioxidant that is required for at least three hundred metabolic functions in the body, including tissue growth and repair, adrenal gland function, and healthy gums. It also aids in the production of anti-stress hormones and interferon, an important immune system protein, and is needed for the metabolism of folic acid, tyrosine, and phenylalanine. Studies have shown that taking Vitamin C can reduce symptoms of asthma, protect against the effects of pollution, helps to prevent cancer, protects against infection, and enhances the immune system. I could go on and on about all the possible benefits of vitamin C. Let me say categorically, this is one vitamin you do not want to be short of.

Sources of Vitamin C are berries, citrus fruits, and green vegetables. Alcohol, analgesics, antidepressants, oral contraceptives, and steroids reduce levels of vitamin C in the body. Smoking causes a serious depletion of this vitamin. It would appear that taking in more vitamin C could help alleviate this problem, but it would be a lot wiser to just stop smoking!

A note of caution regarding taking Vitamin C and aspirin together in large doses is that they can cause stomach irritation leading to ulcers. It has also been found that chewable vitamin C can cause damage to tooth enamel. There is a new version of vitamin C called "Ester C", and it is easier on the stomach lining and more easily utilized by the

---

[11] Ibid, 19

body. It costs a little more, but in my opinion it is well worth the extra expense.

At his annual checkup Bob was given an excellent bill of health. "It must run in your family," said the doctor. "How old was your dad when he died?"

"What makes you think he's dead?" asked Bob. "He's 90 and still going strong."

"Aha! And how long did your grandfather live?" "What makes you think he's dead, Doc? He's 106 and getting married to a 22 year old next week," Bob informed him.

"At his age!" exclaimed the doctor. "Why's he want to marry such a young woman?"

"Doc," replied Bob, "what makes you think he wants to?"

Bioflavonoids: are not true vitamins in the strictest sense and they are sometimes referred to as vitamin P. Bioflavonoids are essential for the absorption of Vitamin C and should be taken together. Some of the various bioflavonoids are: citrin, eriodictyol, flavones, hesperetin, hesperidin, quercetin, quercetrin, and rutin. The human body cannot produce this nutrient, so we must put these in our diet. They are used in the treatment of athletic injuries because they can relieve pain, bruises, and can reduce pain located in legs or across the back.

Working together with Vitamin C, bioflavonoids protects and preserves the structure of capillaries. Quercetin, one of the bioflavonoids, has been shown to be effective in treating and preventing asthma symptoms. Quercetin and bromelain (a digestive enzyme that comes from pineapple that works in conjunction with quercetin) has shown promise in the reduction of allergy symptoms and inflammation.

Natural sources of these nutrients are peppers, buckwheat, black currents, and the white material just beneath the peel of citrus fruits, apricots, blackberries, cherries, grapefruit, grapes, lemons, oranges, plums, and rose hips.

Vitamin D: is a fat-soluble vitamin that has properties of both a vitamin and a hormone, is required for the absorption and utilization of calcium and phosphorus. It is necessary for growth, and is especially important for the normal growth and development of bones and teeth in children. It protects against muscle weakness and is involved in regulation of the heartbeat. It is also important in the prevention and treatment of breast and colon cancer, osteoarthritis, osteoporosis, hypocalcemia, enhances immunity, and is necessary for thyroid function and normal blood clotting.

Sources of Vitamin D are fish liver oils, fatty saltwater fish, dairy products, and eggs. It is also found in butter, cod liver oil, dandelion greens, egg yolks, halibut, liver, milk, oatmeal, salmon, sardines, sweet potatoes, tuna, and vegetable oils. Vitamin D is formed by the body in response to the action of sunlight on the skin. One should always take calcium with Vitamin D

Vitamin E: is an antioxidant that is important in the prevention of cancer and cardiovascular disease. It improves circulation, is necessary for tissue repair, and is useful in treating premenstrual syndrome and fibrocystic disease of the breast. As an antioxidant it prevents cell damage by inhibiting the oxidation of lipids and the formation of free radicals. It is useful in so many beneficial areas that whole books are written about this vitamin alone. For the over fifty group it is an essential addition to your supplement regime.

Sources of Vitamin E are cold pressed vegetable oils, dark green leafy vegetables, legumes, nuts, seeds, whole grains, such as brown rice, cornmeal, dulse, eggs, kelp, desiccated liver, milk, oatmeal, organ meats, soybeans, sweet potatoes, watercress, wheat, bladderwrack, dandelion, dong quai, and flaxseed.

Patient: Doctor, I have a serious memory problem. I can't remember anything!

Doctor: So, when did this problem begin?

Patient: What problem?

Coenzyme Q10: is a vitamin like substance found in all parts of the body. It is an extremely powerful antioxidant whose actions resemble that of Vitamin E. This nutrient can be very important to the readers of this book because it has a profound effect on treatment and prevention of cardiovascular disease.

Coenzyme Q10 has the ability to counter histamine, which makes it beneficial to those with allergies, asthma and other respiratory problems. It also has the ability to aid circulation, stimulate the immune system, increase tissue oxygenation and produces anti-aging effects. The reader should also note that this substance declines in the body as we age.

Natural sources are mackerel, salmon, sardines, beef, peanuts, and spinach. .[12]

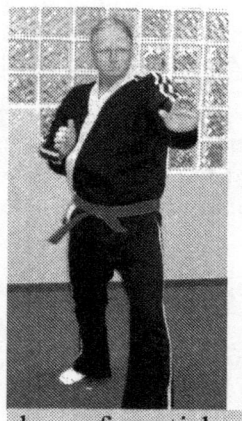

Michael A. is a fifty-five year young building contractor who is extremely healthy, fit and strong for any age. He attributes his current state of wellbeing to spiritual stability, good eating and sleeping habits, stress reduction techniques, consistent exercise and chiropractic care.

He believes people should live to one hundred and he never expects to see a decline in his health or fitness levels. His workout regime consists of four to five days of resistance training and two days of martial arts training. Mike tries to eat mostly organic and

---

[12] Ibid, 23

natural foods, drinks a lot of water and doesn't eat past 7:00 PM. His protein comes from chicken, fish, and a small amount of organic red meat.

Mike doesn't use any pharmaceutical drugs on a regular basis and doesn't smoke or drink alcoholic beverages. He claims to use the following supplements occasionally: antioxidants, garlic, oregano, olive leaf extract, gingko biloba, and omega-3 fatty acids in the form of fish oil.

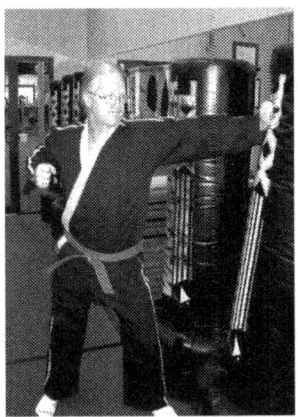

He enjoys reading, researching his interests, and trying to learn new things. His idea of relaxation is to practice martial arts or go to a movie.

Mike has been diagnosed with two herniated disks and has endured shoulder injuries, but he continues to workout wisely under the care of a doctor. He claims that chiropractic adjustments have helped to get relief from pain.

Minerals

Minerals are necessary for the proper composition of body fluids, the formation of blood and bone, the maintenance of healthy nerve function, and the regulation of muscle tone. They act as coenzymes that enable the body to perform its functions, including energy production, growth and healing.

All enzyme activities involve minerals, and they are essential for the proper utilization of vitamins and other nutrients. To get a good look at the amount of minerals, whether or not they are in balance, and the amount of toxic metals in your body, a hair tissue mineral analysis is recommended. This type of analysis can reveal information about minerals, their proper ratios, and levels of toxic metals that go back for the past two months. This will give you a better picture of these things than a blood or urine analysis that lets you know what is going on at that precise moment when the test was taken. Ask your health practitioner about getting one, and if he is not familiar with this procedure, find a naturopath who is.

Let's examine some of the minerals that are needed for our bodies to function properly:

Boron: is needed in trace amounts for healthy bones and muscle growth because it assists in the production of natural steroid compounds within the body. It is also necessary for the metabolism of calcium, phosphorus, and magnesium. It enhances brain function, promotes alertness, and helps in the utilization of energy from fats and sugars. Many people over the age of fifty are deficient in boron.

Boron helps prevent postmenopausal osteoporosis and builds muscle. In a study done by the U. S Department of Agriculture, it showed that supplementing 3 mg. of boron a day for eight days postmenopausal women lost forty percent less calcium, thirty-three percent less magnesium and slightly less phosphorus through their urine than they did prior to supplementing with boron.

Natural sources are found in apples, carrots, grapes, dark green leafy vegetables, pears, whole grains, and raw nuts.[13]

Calcium: is extremely important for the formation of strong bones and teeth, maintenance of healthy gums, maintenance of a regular heartbeat, transmission of nerve impulses, lowers cholesterol levels, and helping prevent cardiovascular disease. For all of these reasons and a few more, calcium is another extremely important mineral for the over fifty group.

Calcium is also needed for muscular growth and contraction, and for the prevention of muscle cramps. A deficiency of this mineral can lead to aching joints, brittle nails, eczema, elevated blood

---

[13] Ibid, 25

cholesterol, heart palpitations, high blood pressure, insomnia, nervousness, rheumatoid arthritis, rickets and tooth decay.

When using a calcium supplement it should be noted that it will have better absorption if taken in smaller doses spread out throughout the day, and taken with magnesium and Vitamin D.

Some of the natural sources of calcium are found in dairy foods, salmon, sardines, seafood, dark leafy vegetables, almonds, cabbage, dulse, figs, filberts, oats, sesame seeds, soybeans, tofu, and many other food sources.

An elderly couple goes to their doctor for a checkup. The man goes in first. "How're you doing?" asks the doctor. "Pretty good," answers the old man. "I'm eating well, and I'm still in control of my bowels and bladder. In fact, when I get up at night to pee, the good Lord turns the light on for me."

The doctor decides not to comment on that last statement, and goes into the next room to check on the man's wife. "How're you feeling?" he asks. "I'm doing well," answers the old woman. "I still have lots of energy and I'm not feeling any pain." The doctor says, "That's nice. It sounds like you and your husband are both doing well.

One thing though - your husband said that when he gets up to pee at night, the good Lord turns the light on for him. Do you have any idea what he means?" "Oh No," says the woman, "He's peeing in the refrigerator again."

Chromium: is involved in the metabolism of glucose, synthesis of cholesterol, fats, and protein. It is important because it maintains stable blood sugar levels through proper insulin utilization. It is important for people with diabetes or hypoglycemia. The average American diet is deficient in chromium.

Chromium deficiencies can lead to anxiety, fatigue, glucose intolerance, inadequate metabolism of amino acids, and an increased risk of arteriosclerosis.

Natural sources of chromium are brewer's yeast, brown rice, cheese, meat, whole grains, calf liver, chicken, eggs, mushrooms, dulse, corn and corn oil, dairy products, and other food or herbal sources.

Copper: aids in the formation of bone hemoglobin and red blood cells, works in balance with zinc and Vitamin C to form elastin (skin protein), works in the healing process, energy production, hair and skin color, and is needed for healthy nerves and joints.

Deficiencies in this mineral can lead to osteoporosis, anemia, baldness, diarrhea, general weakness, impaired respiratory function, and skin sores.

Excessive intake of copper can lead to toxicity and is associated with depression, irritability, nausea and vomiting, nervousness, joint and muscle pain. It should be noted that the level of copper in the body is related to the levels of zinc and Vitamin C.

Natural sources of copper are found in almonds, avocados, barley, beans, beets, blackstrap molasses, broccoli, garlic, lentils, mushrooms, nuts, oats, oranges, pecans, radishes, raisins, salmon, seafood, soybeans, green leafy vegetables, and cookware and plumbing.[14]

Germanium: improves cellular oxygenation and helps to fight pain, keeps the immune system functioning properly and rids the body of toxins.

Natural sources of germanium are broccoli, celery, garlic, shiitake mushrooms, milk, onion, rhubarb, sauerkraut, tomato juice, aloe vera, comfrey and ginseng.

---

[14] Ibid, 28

Iodine: is needed in trace amounts only to help to metabolize excess fat, for physical and mental development, to prevent goiter, and to maintain proper thyroid function. A deficiency in children can result in mental retardation. Certain foods, when eaten in large amounts, will block the uptake of iodine into the thyroid gland. These foods are Brussels sprouts, cabbage, cauliflower, kale, peaches, pears, spinach, and turnips. If you have an under-active thyroid eat these foods in moderation.

Natural sources of iodine are iodized sea-salt, saltwater fish, kelp, asparagus, dulse, garlic, lima beans, mushrooms, sesame seeds, soybeans, spinach, summer squash, and turnip greens.[15]

Iron: is responsible for the production of hemoglobin and myoglobin (the form of hemoglobin found in muscle tissue), and the oxygenation of red blood cells. It is also required for a healthy immune system and for energy production.

Iron deficiency can result from inadequate intake, intestinal bleeding, and a diet high in phosphorus, poor digestion, long term illness, ulcers, prolonged use of antacids, and excessive coffee or tea consumption.

Symptoms of iron deficiency include anemia, brittle hair, difficulty swallowing, digestive disturbances, dizziness, fatigue, fragile bones, hair loss, inflammation of the tissues in the mouth, spoon shaped nails or ridges running lengthwise on the nails, nervousness, obesity, pallor, and slowed mental reactions. Iron is stored in the body and an excess can be a factor involved in such health problems as arthritis, cirrhosis of the liver, diabetes, and heart disorders.

Iron supplements should not be taken unless you are diagnosed with a specific problem that your health provider deems fit to add to your diet.

---

[15] Ibid, 29

Natural sources are eggs, fish, liver, meat, poultry, leafy vegetables, almonds, avocados, kelp, dulse, beets, lentils, millet, kidney and lima beans, pumpkins, soybeans, whole grains, and cereals.

Magnesium: is a vital catalyst in enzyme activity. It is involved in more than four hundred of these activities, especially those activities involving energy production. Magnesium also assists in calcium and potassium uptake. A deficiency can cause the interference of nerve and muscle impulses, and causes irritability and nervousness.

Supplementing the diet with this mineral can help to prevent depression, dizziness, muscle weakness and twitching, premenstrual syndrome, and help maintain the body's proper pH balance and normal body temperature.

In my opinion, magnesium is one of the most important minerals that we should ensure a proper amount of in our daily diet. It is found in many foods, especially dairy products, fish meat and seafood. The consumption of alcohol, the use of diuretics, diarrhea, the presence of fluoride, and high levels of zinc and vitamin D all increase the body's need for magnesium.

Natural sources of magnesium are apples, apricots, avocados, bananas, blackstrap molasses, brewer's yeast, brown rice, cantaloupe, dulse, figs, garlic, grapefruit, green leafy vegetables, kelp, lemons, lima beans, millet, nuts, peaches, black-eyed peas, salmon, sesame seeds, soybeans, tofu, watercress, wheat, and whole grains. [16]

Phosphorus: is needed for blood clotting, bone and tooth formation, cell growth, contraction of the heart muscles, normal heart rhythm, and kidney function. It is also necessary for the body in the utilization of vitamins, and the conversion of food to energy.

Excessive amounts of this mineral can interfere with calcium uptake. This can occur when the diet is high in processed cooked foods and

---

[16] Ibid, 30

junk foods. It is rare to have a deficiency in this mineral because it is found in so many foods.

Natural sources of phosphorus are asparagus, bran, brewer's yeast, corn, dairy products, eggs, fish, dried fruits, garlic, legumes, nuts, sesame, sunflower and pumpkin seeds, meats, poultry, salmon, and whole grains.

"Doctor, are you sure I'm suffering from pneumonia? I heard once about a doctor treating someone with pneumonia and he finally died from typhus."

Don't worry, it won't happen to you with me. If I treat someone with pneumonia, he will die of pneumonia."

Potassium: is important for a healthy nervous system, a regular heart rhythm, helping to prevent stroke, aids in proper muscle contraction, and works with sodium to control the body's water balance.

A deficiency of this mineral can cause dry skin, acne, chills, thinking problems, constipation, depression, diarrhea, diminished reflex function, edema, nervousness, insatiable thirst, fluctuations in heartbeat, glucose intolerance, growth impairment, high cholesterol levels, insomnia, low blood pressure, muscle fatigue and weakness, headaches and salt retention.

Potassium levels can be disrupted by kidney problems, and the use of diuretics or laxatives. Absorption of this mineral can be hampered by tobacco products and by caffeine consumption.

Natural sources of potassium are dairy foods, fish, fruit (apricots, avocados, bananas, figs, and dried fruits such as raisins), legumes, meat, poultry, vegetables, and whole grains (brown rice, and wheat bran). [17]

---

[17] Ibid, 31 - 32

Selenium: has the primary function of inhibiting the oxidation of fats (lipids). It is an extremely important antioxidant, especially when combined with Vitamin E. It protects the immune system, plays a vital role in regulating the effects of thyroid hormone on fat metabolism, and aids in the prevention of tumor formation. It is also important in maintaining a healthy heart and liver, when used in conjunction with Vitamin E.

A deficiency of this mineral has been linked to cancer and heart disease. For this reason alone this mineral becomes very important for the over fifty group. This trace element is needed for pancreatic function and tissue elasticity.

Natural sources of selenium are found in meat, whole grains, Brazil nuts, brewer's yeast, broccoli, chicken, dairy products, dulse, garlic, kelp, salmon, onions, tuna, and wheat germ. [18]

Sodium: is needed to maintain proper water balance and blood pH. It is also necessary for stomach, nerve, and muscle functions. A deficiency of this mineral is rare because it is found in so many sources. You should get your sodium from foods in their natural state; that is, without added salt or salt products.

Balancing sodium with potassium is necessary for good health. When an imbalance exists, heart disease can occur. Due to the fact that most people have too much sodium in their diet, potassium is usually needed in higher amounts to achieve the proper balance.

Zinc: is important for proper prostate gland function, and the growth of reproductive organs. It can help prevent acne by regulating the activity of oil glands; is required for protein synthesis and collagen formation, and promotes a healthy immune system and the healing of wounds.

A deficiency of this mineral can result in the loss of the senses of taste and smell; fingernails can become thin and brittle and develop

---

[18] Ibid, 32

white spots on them. Levels of zinc in the body can be lowered by diarrhea, kidney disease, cirrhosis of the liver, diabetes, or a large consumption of fiber which causes zinc to be extracted through the intestinal tract, and excessive perspiration.

Natural sources of this mineral are brewer's yeast, dulse, egg yolks, fish, kelp, lamb, legumes, lima beans, liver, meats, mushrooms, oysters, pecans, poultry, pumpkin seeds, sardines, seafood, soybeans, sunflower seeds, and whole grains. [19]

Antioxidants/Herbs

Antioxidants are natural substances that will help to protect us against harmful free radicals. In an attempt to give the reader an understanding about what free radicals are, I would say that a free radical cell is one that is missing an electron (normally cells have pairs of electrons) and goes about trying to steal one from another cell; in turn, this other cell now is missing an electron and must go about trying to steal one from another cell. The end result of this can be mutated cells that may become cancerous, -- something we all want to avoid!

Antioxidants help the body by keeping these free radical cells in check by neutralizing them. Obviously this is an over-generalization of a complex process, so we'll examine them just a little closer. Please bear with me, as this is very important information that you will need for your journey.

Free radicals are formed naturally in the body. For example, they are byproducts of normal metabolism, by the breakdown of bacteria by white blood cells, or by enzymatic reactions. They are also formed, in ever-increasing numbers, outside the body by pollution, radiation, cigarette smoke, motor vehicle emissions, and many other processes. These environmental free radicals then enter the body through the

[19] Ibid, 33 - 34

skin, respiration, and other means. Even oxygen, which we need in order to survive, can initiate a free-radical chain reaction in our bodies.

A good example of oxygen free-radical damage can be seen when an apple is sliced in half and left exposed to air. Within a short time, the apple begins to turn brown. This browning is caused by free-radical damage and will eventually destroy the fruit. Whether formed endogenously or exogenously, once in our bodies, these unstable free radicals rob electrons from other molecules to make themselves more stable. In the process, they often cause damage to the body's cells and metabolic processes and many times turn the molecules they have attacked into free radicals themselves. Those molecules, now missing an electron and highly reactive, rob electrons from other molecules, and a chain reaction occurs. This process is called oxidation. It happens all the time in our bodies. In fact, it is estimated that every cell in our body is attacked by free radicals thousands of times a day.

Overall, free radicals have been implicated in the development of at least fifty diseases! A partial list includes arthritis and other inflammatory diseases, kidney disease, cataracts, inflammatory bowel disease, colitis, lung dysfunction, pancreatitis, drug reactions, skin lesions, and aging, to mention a few. Heart disease and cancer are two of the most widespread diseases associated with free radical damage. Heart disease is the leading cause of death in America today, killing an estimated one in every three Americans. Several factors, such as hypertension, cigarette smoking, and diabetes, are the chief culprits in the promotion of heart disease. Literally, free radicals are the major factor of aging, and we are on a journey trying to slow this very process.

Fortunately, the body is able to curb free-radical damage by producing antioxidant molecules and enzymes. Their purpose is to neutralize oxidizing free radicals by donating an electron to them or robbing one from them. The body's arsenal of antioxidants appears to be sufficient for keeping oxidation in check in children and in youths, but once we reach our twenties, the effectiveness of the body's antioxidant defense mechanisms appears to lessen, and free radicals are given greater rein to do damage. The results appear to be, that many of the diseases we associate with aging, including coronary heart disease, cancer, skin damage, Alzheimer's disease, strokes, and rheumatoid arthritis are from free-radical damage. Our prognosis need not be bleak, however. Plants, like humans, produce antioxidants for their own natural defense mechanisms. So, growing all around us are sources of antioxidants that can be ingested to augment our body's natural supply. Indeed, researchers believe that increased dietary intake of antioxidants can slow the process of free-radical damage and associated diseases. Although fruits and vegetables contain the greatest amount of antioxidants in nature, their effectiveness as dietary antioxidants is diminished by two factors: (1) the concentrations of the different types of antioxidants in the plant tissues vary widely, and (2) ripeness, storage, and growing conditions affect these concentrations. For these reasons, it is important to measure the actual antioxidant capacity of fruits, vegetables and dietary antioxidants.

Please do not become overly concerned and begin to worry about this battle between free radicals and antioxidants that is going on in your body on a constant basis. God has made us miraculously, and these processes take place without our knowledge or assistance for the most part. It is when we are exposed to unusual amounts of environmental toxins in the air, in our water, or in our food sources that we must make additional efforts to combat these free radicals.

I've listed herbs and antioxidants together for the simple reason that many herbs are antioxidants. Once again I want to inform you, the reader, to try to get most of your nutrition from the foods and beverages you ingest.

Alpha Lipoic Acid: is a powerful antioxidant that works on its own and as a recycler of Vitamin E and Vitamin C (it can restore the antioxidant properties of these vitamins after they have neutralized free radicals. It also aids and assists the liver, making this supplement one that I highly recommend for everyone over fifty to take on a daily basis.

Bilberry: is a natural antioxidant that helps to keep the walls of the capillary strong and flexible, helps to maintain the flexibility of the walls of red blood cells and allows them to pass through the capillaries easier. This herb also helps to lower blood pressure, inhibits clot formation, enhances blood supply to the nervous system, protects the eyes and may enhance vision, supports and strengthens collagen structure, inhibits growth of bacteria, and has anti-aging and anti-carcinogenic effects. This is another important supplement for the over fifty group that you may want to consider using on a regular basis.

Burdock: possesses powerful antioxidant properties that may protect against cancer by helping to control cell mutation. It has been shown to work best when used in conjunction with Vitamin E.

Carotenoids: See Vitamin A in the previous section on vitamins.

Coenzyme Q10: is an antioxidant that is structurally similar to Vitamin E. It is important for cellular energy production, is an immune system stimulant, can increase circulation, has anti-aging properties, and is important to the cardiovascular system. You may recall that it was previously mentioned under vitamins. Co Q-10 is mentioned twice because of its importance to members of our age group, and this is another supplement that should be considered by everyone reading this book.

Curcumin: is found in the spice turmeric (used in curry and other Indian foods) and has antioxidant properties that prevent the formation of free radicals and neutralize existing free radicals. It stops precancerous changes within DNA and interferes with enzymes necessary for the progression of cancer, stops oxidation of cholesterol, blocks toxic compounds from reaching or reacting with body tissue, and may prevent cataracts.

This herb should not be taken by anyone who is taking anti-coagulants because curcumin acts as a blood thinner.

I don't want to achieve immortality through my work; I want to achieve it through not dying. -- Woody Allen

Flavonoids: are powerful antioxidants and metal chelators. Flavonoids are chemical compounds that are produced by plants for protection from parasites, bacteria, and cell injury. They can be found in fruits, vegetables, spices, seeds, nuts, flowers, and bark. The best sources of Flavonoids are apples, blueberries, bilberries, onions, soy products, and tea.

Garlic: is a miracle herb with many healthful properties. It is a powerful antioxidant, is anti-bacterial, is anti-fungal, is anti-viral, is a potent chelators (helps the body to remove toxins) of toxic heavy metals, can help prevent liver damage, lowers blood pressure, reduces blood cholesterol, and provides protection for the heart. Garlic is a must for every reader to include in his or her diet on a daily basis! You can cook with it, eat it raw, or take in the form of a capsule as a supplement. You can even wear it around your neck to keep vampires away. What more can you ask for?

Gingko Biloba: is a powerful antioxidant that has a strong effect on the brain, retina, and cardiovascular system. It has been used to treat dementia, for long and short term memory improvement, enhances the ability to concentrate, can help with hearing problems, impotence, and macular degeneration.

If you are taking a blood thinning pharmaceutical drug or over-the-counter pain killer you should talk to your health care provider before taking this herb because it can possibly cause internal bleeding.

Grape Seed Extract/Pine Bark Extract (Pycnogenol)/Oligomeric Proanthocyanidins (OPCs): are unique phytochemicals known as Flavonoids that are strong antioxidants that are water soluble and easily absorbed by the body. Studies have shown that they could be as high as fifty times more potent than Vitamin E and twenty times more potent than Vitamin C in terms of bioavailability antioxidant activity.

These antioxidants can protect the brain and spinal nerves against free radical damage, can protect the liver from damage caused by toxic doses of non-prescription pain relievers, and strengthen and repair connective tissue.

Green Tea: possesses antioxidant, anti-bacterial, anti-viral, protect-tion against cancer; lowers cholesterol levels, and possesses other health enhancing properties. It is high in polyphenols because it has not been naturally fermented like black tea. The fermentation process destroys most of the effectiveness as an antioxidant.

Melatonin: is an effective free radical scavenger that can work in all parts of the cell. In laboratory tests it has shown to increase the life span of mice, inhibit cancer growth, stimulate the immune system, and protect against degenerative diseases. It is also effective as a sleep aid when taken just prior to bedtime.

Milk Thistle (Silymarin): protects the liver from toxins and pollutants by preventing free radical damage. Milk thistle can also stimulate the production of new liver cells, and protects the kidneys, is good for gall bladder and adrenal disorders, helps with inflammatory bowel disorders and psoriasis, and has shown anti-cancer effects against prostate cancer and breast cancer. Anyone who has used or abused illegal drugs, prescription drugs, or alcohol in the past or even in the present should utilize this herb on a regular basis.

Selenium: is an essential trace mineral that functions as an antioxidant in conjunction with Vitamin E to protect tissues and cell membranes. Caution should be taken when supplementing with selenium because amounts higher than one milligram taken daily can be toxic.

Vitamin C/Vitamin E/Zinc: See under vitamins or minerals

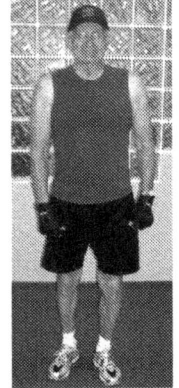

Paul D. is a seventy year young semi-retired building contractor. He is still very active and works out four times per week, and enjoys yard work and boating.

Paul attributes his high level of health and fitness to getting the proper amount of rest everyday, exercising regularly, and eating the right foods. He believes a person should live past ninety, and he doesn't expect to see a decline in his health or fitness levels until he is past ninety.

He walks a mile and a half on a treadmill twice per week and bikes seven miles twice a week. Workouts are generally split by working each body-part twice per week. Paul eats three meals per day and snacks on healthy drinks and energy bars. He doesn't use any tobacco products, drink alcoholic beverages, or take any pharmaceutical drugs on a regular basis.

He supplements his diet with a multi vitamin/mineral, B-12, vitamin

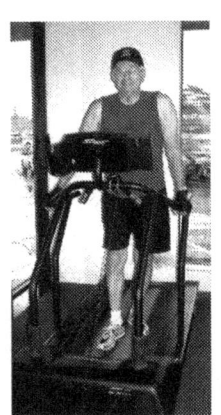

C, and additional protein. His advice for dealing with stress is to simply take a nap. Paul is truly an example of the benefits of a healthy lifestyle. Some years ago Paul was in a four wheeler accident that left him with a severe hip injury. He claims that it was his degree of health and fitness that helped him get through that trying time and to be able to get back to his current levels.

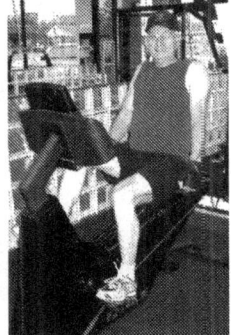

Other Herbs

In the following listing you'll find many of my favorite herbal remedies. Herbal remedies are time tested. Many of them have been used for five thousand years or more. They are used in Chinese medicine, Ayurvedic medicine, American Indian medicine, South American Indian medicine, and by many other people throughout the world. Herbs can be used in the form of essential oils, extracts, powders, salves, ointments, creams, syrups, teas, infusions, decoctions, tinctures, vinegars, and wines. For the average person you will most likely use herbs in capsules, in teas, as seasoning for your food, or as a salve or ointment. You will also find many herbs in shampoos, soaps, and other cosmetics, but it should be noted that these products would have extremely small amounts of helpful herbs.

Modern medicine claims that there is no valid scientific data to support the use of herbs, but the reason there is no such data available is because an herb cannot be patented, copyrighted, or controlled by the pharmaceutical industry or other corporations; thus, there are no profits to be made and expensive testing would be cost prohibitive to small business enterprises.

Many pharmaceutical drugs are actually derived from herbs, where certain components are extracted and are thus eligible for a patent. Examples of some of these drugs are aspirin, which came from the willow tree; digitalis, which comes from the foxglove plant; quinine, which comes from cinchona bark, and others.[20] The only problem in doing this is that there are usually other components of the herb that work in slightly different synergistic ways that either protect us from side effects or enhance the herb's effectiveness.

It should be noted that not all herbs are safe to take while using pharmaceutical drugs when pregnant, or for long periods of time.

---

[20] Ottoboni, Alice & Ottoboni, Fred, (2002) The Modern Nutritional Diseases and how to prevent them, Vincente Books Inc.

You should get recommendations from a knowledgeable person, such as an herbalist, homeopath, or naturopath. The internet also offers lots of information about herbs, but look for websites that are not directly selling these products.

Alfalfa: helps to detoxify the body and helps to raise the body's ph levels. A body that is acidic is usually prone to a variety of sickness and disease. Raising your ph levels generally enhances one's health.

It also has anti-inflammatory, anti-fungal properties; has been found to lower cholesterol, balance blood sugar and hormones, and is good for anemia, arthritis, ulcers, and bone and joint problems. It is a relatively inexpensive herb that I use on a daily basis.

Aloe Vera: works as an astringent, anti-fungal, anti-bacterial, and anti-viral agent. Many people grow their own aloe vera plants and simply break a piece off when needed. I have personally grown and used it on burns with great success. It is also recommended for stomach disorders, but I would caution the reader to buy a ready made juice rather than making your own, unless you have experience in doing so. This herb can be extremely bitter without some processing. Most of the aloe vera products you find in stores today have only a small amount of the herb in it. They are relatively easy to grow, as are most cactus plants.

Black Cohosh: is known to lower cholesterol and blood pressure. It reduced the production of mucus, and aids the cardiovascular and circulatory systems when under stress. This herb is best known for its ability to relieve menopausal symptoms, menstrual cramps associated with back pain, and can help with arthritic conditions.

Boswellia: is an anti-inflammatory, anti-arthritic, anti-fungal, and anti-bacterial agent. It can be used topically to relieve pain. This herb is also useful for liver protection and to help repair blood vessels. I use it daily for its anti-inflammatory properties. Many diseases come about from inflammation, and it is a good idea to protect oneself from it. This herb is well used in Ayurvedic (East Indian) medicine.

Cayenne: will assist digestion, improve one's circulation, and can help to stop the bleeding associated with ulcers. It can aid the immune system in fighting colds, sinus infections, and sore throats. It can be used externally by making a poultice and applying to areas that are painful. It can be used to spice foods, but remember this is a pepper and it can be hot. You must also be careful not to get it on a hot pan because it can emit a gas (similar to a pepper spray) that will cause tearing and discomfort in your eyes. I know this from personal experience!

Joe Bob and Billy Bob, both farmers, met at the state fair.

"Tell me," asked Joe Bob, "what did you give your mule when he had the colic?"

"Turpentine," Billy Bob answered.

A few months after the fair, they meet up again. "Say, Billy Bob, what did you say you gave your mule when he was sick with colic?" Joe Bob asked.

"I said I gave him turpentine."

"Well, I gave turpentine to MINE and it died!"

Billy Bob nods his head. "That's strange. So did mine."

Chamomile: can reduce inflammation, stimulate your appetite, and aid in digestion. It also acts as a tonic that can calm your nerves. It is often used as a tea in combination with other herbs to help with digestion and can help you get relaxed for sleeping.

Cinnamon: is great for regulating glucose in the body, weight loss, relieves diarrhea, nausea, and helps the body eliminate congestion.

It is also known to fight fungal infections. Because it helps the body regulate glucose it is good for people with diabetes. I use it on my oatmeal on a regular basis and it adds a great taste to any cereal. I have also used it on my Ezekiel Bread with olive oil for another tasty treat. Women who are pregnant should be cautioned not to use cinnamon in large amounts.

Cranberry: will acidify urine and prevent bacteria from sticking to bladder cells. It is good for the kidneys, bladder, skin, and has anti-cancer properties. Be careful not to drink cranberry juice drinks that have added sugar. Cranberries are great fresh or dried.

Dandelion: is that pretty little yellow weed growing in your yard that most people try to get rid of. You can eat the leaves (boiled like spinach or in salads), flowers, and even the root can be used. It acts as a diuretic, helps to cleanse the blood and liver, increase bile production, reduce serum cholesterol and uric acid levels. It can also be useful in relieving menopausal symptoms. People taking prescription diuretics should not utilize this herb. One other side note is if you have a pet that may be relieving itself in the yard be sure to wash your herb well before using, or simply buy it from your neighborhood health food store.

Dong Quai: is generally used for menopausal symptoms, premenstrual syndrome, and vaginal dryness. It can act as a mild sedative, laxative, diuretic, and pain reliever. It is quite often found in combination with other herbs that help with female problems.

Echinacea: assists the immune system in fighting bacterial and viral infections. It probably does this by stimulating white blood cells. It is also good for the lymphatic system. People who are allergic to ragweed should not take this herb, and it should not be used by anyone on an ongoing basis. One to two weeks of use when you feel your immune system needs a boost or when you think you have been exposed to a viral or bacterial sickness is all that should be taken.

Elderberry: has been shown to shorten the duration of a bacterial or viral infection and can also limit the symptoms associated with that sickness. It comes in the form of syrup or in capsules. The syrup does not taste bad and is probably better absorbed than the capsules.

Ginger: is great for cooking with when you want to add that special taste that only ginger has. I use it often when making a stir fry dish. It has a calming effect on the stomach, has anti-inflammatory properties, cleanses the colon, reduces spasms and cramps, and can stimulate circulation. Ginger is often given to people on cruise ships to help with motion sickness.

Ginseng: can strengthen the adrenal and reproductive glands, enhance the immune system, and is used by athletes for overall body strengthening. Ginseng has been a sought after herb for thousands of years. It is said that wars have been fought in China over this herb. It is well used in Oriental medicine.

Goldenseal: is a good herb to use in conjunction with Echinacea to support the immune system during stressful times (i.e. when you are exposed to colds and flu viruses). It also fights inflammation, helps to cleanse the body, reduces blood pressure, helps insulin to work more efficiently, and is helpful during allergy season. This herb should not be used for long periods of time, and should be avoided if you have high blood pressure, suffer from insomnia, are pregnant, or are nursing a baby. I recommend seven to ten day periods of use at a time.

Hawthorn: is good for your heart in that it lowers blood pressure, lowers cholesterol levels, reduces levels of fat deposits, dilates coronary blood vessels, and restores heart muscle. It is also useful for people with anemia, circulatory disorders, and a suppressed immune system. This is definitely an herb to consider for the over fifty group.

Hops: work well to relieve anxiety, stimulate the appetite, help achieve a restful sleep, and cardiovascular disorders. You can place this herb inside a pillowcase to help you get a good night sleep. If you are taking an antidepressant do not use this herb.

Lavender: works well to calm a restless person. You can use it as an essential oil and place a few drops on your pillow at night to help you get a good night sleep. It also relieves stress, depression, headaches, skin disorders, and is good for burns.

An old woman came into her doctor's office and confessed to an embarrassing problem. "I fart all the time, Doctor Johnson, but they're soundless, and they have no odor. In fact, since I've been here, I've farted no less than twenty times. What can I do?"

"Here's a prescription, Mrs. Harris. Take these pills three times a day for seven days and come back and see me in a week."

Next week an upset Mrs. Harris marched into Dr. Johnson's office. "Doctor, I don't know what was in those pills, but the problem is worse! I'm farting just as much, but now they smell terrible! What do you have to say for yourself?"

"Calm down, Mrs. Harris," said the doctor soothingly. "Now that we've fixed your sinuses, we'll work on your hearing!!!"

Olive Leaf: is a favorite of mine. I use it year round to ward off allergy problems. It is anti-bacterial, anti-viral, anti-fungal, and helps the body fight off parasites. This herb has shown promise in helping people with chronic fatigue syndrome.

Pau d'Arco: has an anti-bacterial and anti-viral property. It is good for combating a yeast overgrowth, tumors, smoker's cough, and all types of infections. This herb is also used to fight cancer.

Peppermint: aids digestion by increasing stomach acidity, and is useful for most stomach distress. It is easily grown and can be eaten right off the plant. You should be careful using this herb if you are anemic because it may interfere with iron absorption, and it should not be used by nursing mothers.

Primrose: is also called *evening primrose* promotes cardiovascular health, helps reduce the symptoms of menstrual problems, and is helpful in treating alcoholism, arthritis, hot flashes, and skin disorders. This herb, in conjunction with other herbs, is usually recommended for women going through menopausal problems. This herb should not be used during pregnancy.

Pygeum: reduces inflammation and is a natural decongestant. It is useful in treating prostate enlargement by reducing inflammatory compounds found in the prostate.

St. John's Wort: is an excellent alternative for fighting depression and nerve pain. In many European countries this herb is prescribed more often than any pharmaceutical antidepressant. It has been found to be most effective when used in conjunction with 5-HTP, and magnesium. This herb is also known to protect bone marrow and intestinal mucosa from x-ray damage. When used in the form of oil, it assists in wound healing. It should be noted that large amounts of this herb can cause sun sensitivity, and should not be used by people taking prescription antidepressants.

Saw Palmetto: is most often used in prevention of prostate enlargement. It acts as a diuretic, urinary antiseptic, and appetite stimulant. It is often used in Europe to treat benign prostate hyperplasia.

Tea Tree: is commonly found in soap, shampoo, and topical solutions. It disinfects wounds and has a healing effect on most skin conditions (i.e. acne, athlete's foot, boils, cuts, scrapes, fungal infections, herpes outbreaks, scalp problems, insect and spider bites, and warts). You can use this herb to make a solution to gargle that is effective for healing sore throats, colds, and mouth sores. If used internally it should be diluted or distilled.

Valerian: is useful in treating insomnia, anxiety, fatigue, high blood pressure, irritable bowel syndrome, nervousness, pain, spasms, stress, ulcers, menstrual and muscle cramps. It can be found and used in herbal sleep formulas, or individually.

White Willow Bark: contains the compounds that are found in aspirin, and is useful for relieving pain, allergies, headaches, backaches, nerve pain, point pain, inflammation, menstrual cramps, and toothaches. It is safer to use this herb than aspirin, but should not be taken if you are allergic to aspirin.

Wild Yam: is good for reducing inflammation, relaxing muscle spasms, and promotes perspiration. It contains compounds that are similar to the hormone progesterone. This herb has been used successfully in treating colic, gallbladder disorders, hypoglycemia, irritable bowel syndrome, kidney stones, and female disorders such as premenstrual syndrome, and menopause related conditions.

Witch Hazel: is used topically and is good for relieving itching, mouth and skin inflammation, and symptoms associated with hemorrhoids. I use witch hazel as an effective after shave solution.

Yohimbe: is known to increase blood flow to the male sex organ and may increase levels of the male hormone testosterone. Caution should be used when using this herb because it can possibly induce anxiety, panic attacks, and hallucinations in some people.

Amino Acids

Amino Acids are the chemical units that make up proteins. They are commonly referred to as "Building blocks", and are the end production of protein digestion. Amino Acids are extremely important because they are essential to life. Often these nutrients are overlooked as aids in restoring our body to a healthy state.

They are different from carbohydrates and fats in that they contain nitrogen and the others do not. All living organisms are composed of protein, and protein participates in the vital chemical processes that maintain life.

Supplemental forms of amino acids are available, and I want the reader to be informed about the various benefits you could derive from them. They come in a variety of forms, free form being the purest form that requires no digestion and can be digested directed into the bloodstream. The "L form" of amino acids are more compatible with our biochemistry.

Amino Acids should not be taken for long periods of continuous use. A general rule about amino acid supplementation is to alternate the individual amino acid with an amino acid complex for two months on and two months off in intervals.

I will list the amino acids that I feel could be the most benefit to people that are "middle aged," meaning people who are fifty to one hundred years young.

Alanine: plays an important role in the transfer of nitrogen from peripheral tissue to the liver. It assists in the metabolism of glucose, and guards against the buildup of toxic substances that are released in muscle cells.

Arginine: slows the growth of tumors and cancer by enhancing the immune system. It is capable of increasing the size of the thymus gland, which manufactures "T-Cells" which are crucial parts of the immune system.

This amino acid may be beneficial to those with AIDS and malignant diseases that suppress the immune system. It is also effective in use for people with liver disorders and is said to aid the liver in the detoxification process by neutralizing ammonia. It is important for muscle metabolism, can reduce the effects of alcohol toxicity, is helpful in the repair of damaged tissue, and may be helpful in treating men who are sterile.

Natural sources of this amino acid are carob, chocolate, dairy products, gelatin, meat, oats, peanuts, soybeans, walnuts, wheat and wheat germ.

People with viral infections such as herpes should not take supplemental Arginine and should avoid the foods that are rich in it. Others who should avoid supplementing this amino acid are pregnant or lactating women, and schizophrenics.

Alice is terribly overweight, so her doctor puts her on a diet. "I want you to eat regularly for two days, then skip a day, and repeat this procedure for two weeks. The next time I see you, you'll have lost at least five pounds."

When Alice returns, she's lost nearly 20 pounds. "Wow, that's amazing!!" the doctor says. "Did you follow my instructions?"

She nods. "I'll tell you, though; I thought I was going to drop dead that third day." "From hunger, you mean?" asked the doctor.

"No, from skipping."

Aspartic Acid: is good for fighting fatigue and depression, increases one's stamina, plays a vital role in metabolism, is beneficial for people with neural and brain disorders, is good for athletes, and aids the liver by removing excess ammonia and helps the body to remove other toxins.

Plant protein found in sprouted seeds contains an abundance of this amino acid. This amino acid plus phenylalanine are used to make the artificial sweetener aspartame. This sweetener should be avoided at all cost, in like fashion to other villains that are trying to take you out. Aspartame is what is known as an "excitotoxin," and they are known to destroy brain neurons for up to two hours after ingestion. Diseases such as Alzheimer's, ALS and other neuro-muscular diseases have been associated to its use.

Carnitine: is a substance that is very similar to a B-Vitamin. It is useful in transporting long chain fatty acids that are used to provide energy within the cells. Because of this, it is apparent that it will increase the use of fats for cellular energy, and possibly prevent the buildup of fat in the body. This substance may be useful in treating chronic fatigue syndrome, diabetes, lower blood triglycerides, and can be helpful for those trying to lose weight. Carnitine can enhance the effectiveness of antioxidants and may slow the aging process. It requires an adequate level of Vitamin C to synthesize this substance. Acetyl L Carnitine has been shown to slow the progression of Alzheimer's disease and has a positive effect on depression.

Cysteine & Cystine: are two amino acids that are closely related, and each is capable of converting to L-cystine. They are sulfur containing and aid in the formation of skin and are very important in the process of detoxification.

Cysteine can help to detoxify harmful toxins and give the user protection from radiation damage. When taken with selenium and Vitamin E it is an excellent free radical destroyer. Supplementing with L-cysteine has been found to be useful in treating rheumatoid arthritis, hardening of the arteries, and even cancer. It can help the body's process of repairing burned tissue, and will chelate heavy metals (aiding in detoxification).
N-acetyl cysteine (NAC) may be used in place of L-cysteine, and will aid in preventing some of the side effects from chemotherapy or radiation therapy. This amino acid also has anti-aging benefits for the body in that it reduces the accumulation of age spots, and all of the other benefits mentioned for cysteine.

This is definitely a supplement that anyone over fifty should consider utilizing. The only exception would be for anyone with diabetes, who should be careful when considering supplementing with cysteine because it may inactivate insulin.

Gamma-Aminobutyric Acid (GABA): acts as a neurotransmitter in the central nervous system. It is crucial for metabolism in the brain, thus aiding the brain to function properly

This amino acid can be used to calm the body, in much the same way as diazepam (Valium), or other tranquilizers without the fear of addiction or harmful side effects. It is also useful in treatment of epilepsy and hypertension, and is also useful in treating people with a depressed sex drive and enlarged prostate.

When supplementing with GABA be careful not to overdo it because it can cause shortness of breath, numbness around the mouth, and tingling in the extremities. It is always a good idea to consult with a health care practitioner before use of most supplementation.

Glutamic Acid: is an important amino acid that helps the body to metabolize sugars and fats. It also assists in the transportation of potassium into the spinal fluid and across the brain barrier. This amino acid can also be converted to glutamine or GABA.

It has been shown helpful in correcting personality disorders and for treating childhood behavioral disorders. It is also useful in the treatment of epilepsy, mental retardation, muscular dystrophy, ulcers, and hypoglycemic coma.

Glutamine: is the most abundant free amino acid found in the muscles of the human body, and is also known as brain fuel. It is extremely important in that it helps the body to regulate the proper acid and alkaline balance in the body. It is highly recommended to people who have digestive problems, and it also promotes mental ability. In supplement form it can be helpful in treating arthritis, autoimmune disease, fibrosis, intestinal disorders, peptic ulcers, connective tissue disease, impotence, depression, senility, and other mental disorders. It should be avoided by persons who suffer from cirrhosis of the liver or kidney problems.

Cooking can destroy this amino acid, so it is best absorbed when eating raw spinach and parsley.

Glutathione: is not technically an amino acid, but is produced by the body from the amino acids cysteine, Glutamic acid, and Glycine.

Glutathione is a powerful antioxidant produced by the liver, where it works to detoxify harmful compounds that can be excreted through the bile. The best way to help the body produce this amino acid is by supplementing N-acetyl cysteine (NAC).

Glycine: slows muscle degeneration by supplying creatine, which assists in the construction of DNA and RNA. It is interesting to note that having the proper amount of this amino acid in your system helps to produce energy, but when there is an excess of this amino acid it can do the exact opposite and cause fatigue.

This amino acid is important in maintaining a healthy prostate, and in the treatment of manic depression, and hyperactivity disorder.

Histidine: is an important amino acid that assists the body in growth and repair of tissue, aids in the maintenance of myelin sheaths, which protect nerve cells, assist the body in the production of red and white blood cells; protects the body from radiation damage, helps to lower blood pressure, aids in the removal of heavy metals from the body, and may help to prevent AIDS.

When levels of this amino acid are too high, it can lead to stress and anxiety, and possibly schizophrenia. When the levels of this amino acid drop too low, it may contribute to rheumatoid arthritis. So, you see how important it is to have the correct level of this and other nutrients in our body.

This amino acid should not be taken in supplements by persons suffering from manic depression.

This elderly couple is watching one of those television preachers on TV one night. The preacher faces the camera, and announces,

"My friends, I'd like to share my healing powers with everyone watching this program. Place one hand on top of your TV & the other hand on the part of your body which ails you & I will heal you."

The old woman has been having terrible stomach problems, so she places one hand on the television, and her other hand on her stomach. Meanwhile, her husband approaches the television, placing one hand on top of the TV and his other hand on his groin.

With a frown his wife says, "Ernest, he's talking about healing the sick, not raising the dead."

Isoleucine: is an essential amino acid responsible for stabilizing blood sugar and energy levels, and is needed for the formation of hemoglobin. A deficiency of this amino acid can lead to symptoms similar to those of hypoglycemia.

Good food sources of this amino acid are almonds, cashews, chicken, chickpeas, eggs, fish, lentils, liver, meat, rye, most seeds, and soy protein.

Leucine: is one of the branched chain amino acids. The others are Isoleucine and Valine. They work synergistically to protect muscle tissue, act as a fuel, and promote the healing of bones, skin, and muscle tissue. This amino acid is often recommended for people recovering from surgery.
Natural sources of Leucine are brown rice, beans, nuts, soy flour, and whole wheat.

Lysine: is necessary as a building block for all protein, and is needed for growth and bone development in children. For the over fifty group it could be used for sports injury and surgical recoveries; and is useful when fighting cold sores, and the herpes viruses.

It has been found that supplementing with this amino acid, Vitamin C and bioflavonoids can effectively fight and prevent herpes outbreaks.

Deficiencies of this amino acid can result in anemia, blood shot eyes, hair loss, concentration problems, fatigue, irritability, poor appetite, and lack of growth.

Methionine: helps in the breaking down of fats and helps to prevent their buildup in the liver and arteries. It also helps the digestive system by detoxifying harmful agents such as lead and other heavy metals.

This amino acid is a powerful antioxidant and a good source of sulfur, which helps to prevent skin and nail problems. Natural sources are beans, eggs, fish, garlic, lentils, meat, onions, soybeans, seeds and yogurt. The supplements choline and lecithin can be used to add methionine to the diet.

Ornithine: helps the body to release growth hormones which aid in the metabolism of fat. This effect can be enhanced by adding Arginine and Carnitine with it. This amino acid is necessary for the immune system and liver to function properly.

Supplemental L-ornithine should not be taken by children, pregnant women, nursing mothers, or people with a history of schizophrenia.

Phenylalanine: has a direct effect on brain chemistry by synthesizing two key neurotransmitters that promote alertness: dopamine and norepinephrine. It can help to elevate mood, decrease pain sensations, assist in memory and learning, and even suppress the appetite. It could be quite helpful for those struggling with weight problems.

Pregnant women, people who suffer from anxiety attacks, have diabetes, high blood pressure, skin cancer, or PKU should not take phenylalanine in supplemental form.

Proline: improves the texture of one's skin by assisting in the production of collagen and reducing the loss of collagen through the aging process. It can also strengthen joints, tendons, and the heart muscle. It can be obtained by eating meat, dairy products, and eggs.

Serine: is necessary for proper metabolism of fats and fatty acids, the growth of muscle, and maintenance of our immune system. An excessive amount of this amino acid can have a negative effect on our immune system, so we should ingest the foods listed below in moderation.

Natural sources of serine are meat, soy products, dairy foods, gluten, and peanuts. Unfortunately many of these foods cause an allergic reaction in the some of us.

Taurine: can be helpful for people with atherosclerosis, edema, heart disorders, hypertension, and hypoglycemia. It is needed for the proper utilization of sodium, potassium, calcium, and magnesium. Taurine is found in eggs, fish, meat, and milk.

Doctor: You're in good health. You'll live to be eighty.

Patient: But, doctor, I am 80 right now.

Doctor: See, what did I tell you.

Threonine: helps to maintain the proper balance of protein in the body, and is important in the formation of collagen, elastin, and tooth enamel. This amino acid also aids the immune system and may be helpful in treating some types of depression.

Trytophan: is the amino acid that became infamous in the late 1980s when it was found that some contaminated batches of this supplement were linked to several hundred cases of eosinophiliamyalgia syndrome (EMS). It was later determined that the contaminated supplement, not the Trytophan, was the likely culprit in the cases of EMS.

To this date, Trytophan is still banned from the market in the United States. If pharmaceutical drugs were banned when they caused the same approximate number of problems as did the Trytophan supplement, we would have very few pharmaceutical drugs on the market today.

This amino acid is utilized by the brain to produce serotonin (the feel good hormone that helps to regulate mood and sleep patterns). 5-HTP, which comes from Trytophan, is sold over the counter and can help to build serotonin, and produce similar results as the amino acid produces. I believe the combination of St. John's Wort, magnesium, and 5-HTP work well synergistically to help combat depression, without the harmful side effects of many of the SSRI's that are prescribed today.

Trytophan can be found in brown rice, cottage cheese, meat, peanuts, turkey, and soy protein.

Tyrosine: helps the body maintain its overall metabolic rate. It is useful as a mood elevator and to combat depression; suppresses the appetite, and helps to reduce body fat.

The L-form of this amino acid has been used for stress reduction, and it may be helpful in combating chronic fatigue and narcolepsy.

Natural sources are almonds, avocados, bananas, dairy products, lima beans, pumpkin seeds, and sesame seeds. People taking an MAO for depression must strictly limit their intake of these types of food containing tyrosine, or any supplements with it.

Valine: is needed for muscle metabolism, tissue repair, to help the body maintain a proper balance of nitrogen. It may be helpful in treating liver and gall bladder disease.

Valine can be found in dairy products, grains, meat mushrooms, peanuts, and soy protein. It should be taken in balance with other branch chain amino acids when used in supplemental forms.

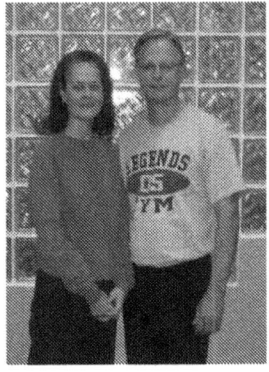

Bob N. is a fifty-four year young entrepreneur who looks years younger than his chronological age. His spouse, Ava S., is also outlined in this book. They are truly a health and fitness couple, and as you can see, it is quite helpful when both partners share similar health and fitness views.

Bob attributes his present state of health and fitness to "clean living." He doesn't smoke or drink, exercises regularly, watches what he eats, limits his sugar intake, and avoids fried foods.

Bob eats three times per day, and eats some fruit between meals. In the morning he drinks coffee and a glass of pure fruit juice along with his cereal. For lunch and dinner he eats low fat, non-fried foods which include chicken, turkey, fish and a small amount of beef. He also includes the following supplements into his dietary regime: Multi vitamin/mineral, vitamin E, vitamin C, calcium, and protein drinks.

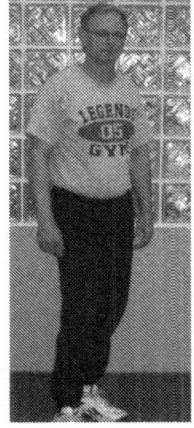

His workouts consist of a four day split routine where he works each body-part two times per week, and he does cardio four times a week as well. Occasionally Bob experiences some "burnout" from his fitness regime, so he takes off for a week or two and then gets back to working out again, or he makes some changes to his routine.

When asked how long a person should live, he responded with one hundred and fifty years, but he did state that he has seen a decline in his health and fitness levels already. The reader should understand that he or she may not be able to perform at the same level you have when in your twenties or thirties, but you can maintain a high degree of fitness regardless. This is an important point for the over fifty group to understand.

Other Supplementation

I've included this listing of supplements that I feel are important for the over fifty group. Always remember that not all supplements are beneficial to all people. Due to the fact that we all have a unique physiology, it is always best to discuss your health needs with a qualified health care professional.

Chondroitin Sulfate: helps to create cartilage, and has been shown to attract and maintain water in joint cartilage. The supplemental form is usually derived from powdered shark cartilage or cow trachea cartilage, and is helpful in the treatment of osteoarthritis.

It is usually recommended to take chondroitan sulfate along with glucosamine, and oftentimes with the addition of MSM to make a powerful therapy in treating joint problems. I have read many studies on the use of these supplements to treat joint problems, and it appears as though these supplements help in approximately fifty percent of the people using them. This means it doesn't work for everyone. My advice would be to give it a try and see if it works for you.

You should use caution in taking chondroitan sulfate if you are taking any type of blood thinner, because it is chemically similar to the blood thinner heparin. Pregnant women should also avoid using this supplement due to the lack of sufficient studies to indicate its safety during this time.

Creatine: has been shown to increase strength and endurance. It is quite popular with athletes because it allows them to work out harder and make greater gains. It has also been shown to make muscles appear fuller.

I have noted that using creatine regularly has a positive effect on prevention of back pain. This may occur because of the addition of fluid to muscle giving the joints and spinal disks more protection.

Whenever supplementing with creatine you should be sure to get plenty of fresh water every day because creatine may place stress on the kidneys.

DHEA: is a hormone produced mainly by the adrenal glands, and is important in the production of testosterone, progesterone, and corticosterone. Unfortunately DHEA production declines with age, particularly after the age of forty.

There has been research that shows supplementing with DHEA may prevent cancer, arterial disease, multiple sclerosis, and Alzheimer's disease. You should use caution when supplementing with DHEA because when taken in high dosage it may suppress your own production of this vital hormone, and it can even make it difficult for your body to synthesize.

Possible side effects of taking DHEA may be excess growth of facial hair for women. Another alternative is to take 7-Keto DHEA which is not converted to estrogen or testosterone, and may have all of the other benefits. It is a good idea to talk to your health care practitioner before using this supplement.

Fish Oil: is a great source of omega-3 fatty acids. Omega-3 fatty acids have been found to be effective in the treatment of heart and circulatory system problems, chronic pain syndrome, arthritic conditions, and joint problems. When taking as a supplement it should be noted that doses of more than two grams per day may have a harmful amount of PCP's, dioxin, or mercury, but you can purchase pharmaceutical grade fish oil that removes 99.9% of these toxins. Because it may be called pharmaceutical grade does not mean it has to be purchased from a pharmacy. You can find this product in most health food stores.

These same toxins (that may be found in non-pharmaceutical grade fish oil) can be found in farm raised fish, and fish caught in certain parts of the world. Natural sources of fish oil are wild salmon, mackerel, herring, and sardines.

I personally recommend pharmaceutical grade fish oil for all persons in the over fifty group. If you are taking it strictly for preventative measures, two grams per day is usually adequate, but if you are treating sickness or disease, a higher dose is usually required. See your health care provider for guidance in the correct dosage for you to use.

Flaxseed Oil/Flaxseed: is another rich source of omega-3 fatty acids. It also contains magnesium, potassium, fiber, B vitamins, protein and zinc. Flaxseed makes a good addition to salads, soup, cereals, yogurt, or baked goods. A problem that I personally encounter with the use of flaxseed is that they get stuck beneath the gum line and between teeth. I like to alternate the use of fish oil and flaxseed oil taken with each meal on a daily basis. All of the benefits of omega-3 fatty acids that are in fish oil also apply to flaxseed oil.

Glucosamine: is involved in the formation of nails, tendons, skin, eyes, bones, ligaments, and heart valves. It is found in high concentrations in joint structures. As a supplement, glucosamine sulfate is helpful in dealing with symptoms of osteoarthritis, and other joint problems. It has been shown that glucosamine actually helps to build joint cartilage. Most supplements that are effective contain glucosamine sulfate, chondroitan sulfate, and MSM.

Research indicates that the use of glucosamine and chondroitan are helpful for over fifty percent of the people who try it for thirty days or more.

5-HTP: is a substance that is derived from the amino acid Trytophan. The body can use this substance to create serotonin, an important neurotransmitter. In Germany and other European countries, the most often used prescription for depression is be St. John's Wort, 5-HTP, and magnesium taken three times per day. Always remember that you should not use this type of supplementation if you are already taking any type of SSRI.

Discuss taking this supplement with your health care practitioner prior to use.

Kelp: is a type of seaweed which is a rich source of B-vitamins, minerals (especially iodine), and many trace elements. It can be eaten raw, granulated and used as a seasoning, and liquid form. It has been found to be useful in treating thyroid conditions, hair loss problems, nail disorders, obesity and ulcers. It can also protect from radiation, and soften stools.

The iodine in the kelp can help a person rev up their metabolism by stimulating the thyroid gland.

Mushrooms: The following mushrooms taste good and are excellent for boosting the immune system and for other listed benefits:
- *Maitake:* helps the body to adapt to stress, normalizes bodily functions, inhibits the growth of cancerous tumors, enhances the activity of important immune cells, and may be useful in the treatment of chronic fatigue syndrome, obesity, and high blood pressure.
- *Shiitake:* contains seven essential amino acids, and eleven other amino acids. It is rich in B-vitamins, and has high amounts of vitamin D. It has been shown to be effective in cancer treatment, and it strengthens the immune system.

80

- *Reishi:* has been used in Chinese medicine for centuries and is believed to enhance longevity. It is also used to treat high blood pressure, heart disease, cholesterol problems, fatigue, and viral infections.
- *Cordyceps:* has also been shown to be effective in treating disorders that require a boost to the immune system for treatment.

These and other types of mushrooms are all excellent additions to one's diet. You can cook them with eggs, stir fry dishes, and use in casseroles. They are also excellent in salads. You can also get them in a capsule for those that do not like the taste of mushrooms. The over fifty group members should consider using them regularly.

MSM: is a naturally occurring organic sulfur compound found in plants and animal tissue. It has been found to nourish hair, skin, and nails, and has been proven to relieve pain and inflammation. Due to its ability to reduce pain, it is often used in conjunction with glucosamine and chondroitan for joint problems.

It has also been found to enhance immune function, benefit those suffering from heartburn, arthritis, lung problems, and migraine headaches.

Natural sources of MSM are fresh fish, meats, plants, fruit, and milk. Processing of foods eliminate most of the MSM content they once possessed. Because of this fact supplementation is recommended by taking approximately one gram two times per day. As with most supplements, you should give your body a break-in period where you gradually increase the dosage until you reach the desired dose without any undesirable affects.

Probiotics: are the friendly bacteria found in the digestive system. In my opinion everyone should take a supplemental probiotic daily. It will serve as an important part of the digestive process, help to prevent yeast overgrowth and other pathogens, and assist in the synthesis of Vitamin K. Whenever a person takes in antibiotics it destroys all the bacteria in your body. That includes the good bacteria as well as the harmful, and this is the reason many doctors will tell their patients to take probiotics after a round of antibiotics. By increasing your friendly bacteria count you will give your immune system a boost as well as the other benefits mentioned.

Natural sources of friendly bacteria are cultured or fermented foods such as buttermilk, yogurt, cheese, kefir, miso, sauerkraut, tempeh, and umeboshi. The miso, tempeh, and umeboshi are used in Japanese cuisine.

Progesterone Cream: can help women who are estrogen dominant to balance their hormones in a natural way with few, if any, side effects. In the over fifty group you are most likely in a peri menopausal, or menopausal state. This simply means you are going through a natural change in your life where you will cease to have monthly periods, and when your body will produce less estrogen at this time.

Progesterone cream, when used in a proper dose (which is the amount that your body should normally produce) can help to eliminate some of those unpleasant side effects of your body adjusting its hormonal state. I recommend that you get a saliva test to find out exactly what your hormonal state is, and then under the care of a knowledgeable health care provider use whatever natural hormones your body needs to balance itself.

When purchasing progesterone creams make sure that the bottle lists an amount of natural progesterone contained in that bottle (i.e. 400mg – 900mg per bottle). The reason I say this is because there are some progesterone creams out there that have very little useable progesterone or no progesterone in it.

SAMe: is derived from the amino acid methionine. It has been shown to have a positive effect on depression, joint problems, connective tissue disorders, liver health, and cardiovascular disease.

SAMe should always be taken on an empty stomach. Anyone with manic-depressive disorder should consult with their health care practitioner before using this supplement.

Whey Protein: is excellent source of amino acids that will assist your body in building lean body mass. It is an excellent way of balancing your meals that are deficient in protein. I like to put a scoop (which contains approximately twenty grams of protein) in my morning cereal, and I like to mix it with soy milk to make a great tasting muscle building drink.

Other benefits of whey protein are the protection from muscle-wasting in people with AIDS or cancer; it appears to inhibit to growth of cancer cells, and it protects the body from free radical damage.

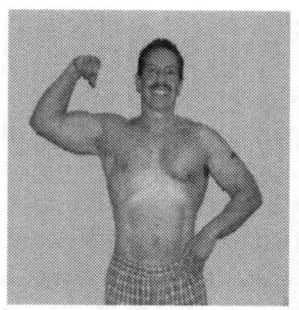

My Personal Supplement Regime

Whole Food Multi Vitamin/Mineral: I take one per day. The recommended dose is three per day, but I get many valuable nutrients by eating well and supplementing other individual vitamins and minerals. I feel as though I really do not need any more.

Full Spectrum Minerals: Tablet taken once per day in the morning.

Ester C w/Bioflavonoids: 500 mg. taken two times per day (one in the morning and one at night).

B-Complex: high dose of all of the B Vitamins taken once per day (in the morning).

Probiotics: Capsule taken twenty minutes prior to eating in the morning.

Vitamin E: 400 IU taken once per day (at night).

Calcium/Magnesium: 1000mg/500mg taken in two capsules (morning and night).

Magnesium: 200 mg. taken at bedtime.

Fish Oil: 1000 mg. taken twice per day (one after breakfast and one after dinner).

Flax Seed Oil: 1000 mg. taken twice per day (one after lunch and one at night).

Creatine Monohydrate: one teaspoon per day, or two capsules in the morning and night.

Whey Protein: Mixed in cereal every morning and in a drink after workouts.

Alpha Lipoic Acid: 100 mg. taken twice per day (morning and night).

Olive Leaf Extract: Capsules taken twice per day (morning and night).

Bromelain: 500 mg. taken twice per day (morning and night).

DHEA: 25 mg. taken on occasion when I feel I need a little extra strength and I take it once per day (morning).

Kelp: Capsules taken twice per day (morning and evening).

Ginger: Capsules taken twice per day (morning and night).

Alfalfa: Capsules taken twice per day (morning and night).

Boswellin: Capsules taken when an additional anti-inflammatory agent is needed and is taken once per day.

Milk Thistle: I take these on an irregular basis (four to six week intervals) for three days (two capsules per day).

Mushroom Combination: Capsules are taken when I feel a need to boost my immune system.

Please refer to the section on supplementation to get a full understanding about how these supplements are beneficial.

Exercise

Setting a goal is not the main thing.
It is deciding how you will go about achieving it and staying with that plan.
Tom Landry (Dallas Cowboys Coach)

Exercise is an important component of maintaining and achieving health. Our bodies are designed for movement. Without this movement we cannot function optimally. Muscles begin to shrink (called atrophy) when not used, and bone density decreases when our body's structure is not taxed. Our internal organs do not function well when the body is not being moved. There are many ways to achieve health through a variety of bodily movements, but I do want to emphasize it is extremely important to so on a regular basis. As we age it is more important to exercise on a daily basis! For myself I have noticed that I have far fewer aches, pains or discomforts when I exercise daily.

Like muscle, bone is living tissue that responds to exercise by becoming stronger. Women and men who exercise regularly generally achieve greater peak bone mass (maximum bone density and strength) than those who do not. For most people, bone mass peaks during the third decade of life. After that time, we can begin to lose bone. Women and men older than age twenty can help prevent bone loss with regular exercise.

Exercising allows us to maintain muscle strength, coordination, and balance, which in turn helps to prevent falls and related fractures. This is especially important for older adults and people who have been diagnosed with osteoporosis.

Many people confuse exercise with work, especially hard work. First of all I want to state that no matter what type of work you do, you should still exercise regularly. As we have reached the beginning phases of middle age (remember that is fifty to one hundred years of age) most of us do not work as hard physically as we may have in the past. At this stage of life many of us have been placed in supervisory positions where we leave the harder work to the twenty and thirty year olds. Also bear in mind that there is a different mindset used during exercise than the one used during work, and this also makes a huge difference in the way our bodies respond to this type of movement.

Exercise is essential for health and will be discussed in detail in the chapter on fitness. Be sure to read the entire section on fitness prior to starting any new or additional programs.

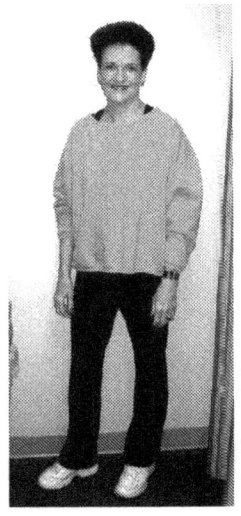

Jan L. has worked in the fitness industry for many years. Currently she teaches an aerobics class three times per week, and a senior's fitness class twice per week. Jan is a vibrant, healthy and fit woman, who at the age of fifty-nine, appears to be many years younger.

She attributes her good health and fitness level to "consistent dedication to exercise, proper nutrition, an ability to handle stress, and a positive attitude".

Jan eats at least ninety grams of protein, two to three fruits, two to three servings of green vegetables, and organic yogurt as her daily staples. She takes a moderate amount of whole food supplements and extra calcium daily.

Her relationship with God is "very good," and she continually works on improving it.

Sleep

Early to bed and early to rise, makes a man healthy, wealthy, and wise.
Benjamin Franklin

You hear so many concepts about the right amount of sleep. I think the amount of sleep a person should get depends on the requirements of each person individually. Some people require eight hours per night, while others require ten hours per night, and still others may require only six hours. The best way to judge the correct amount of sleep for yourself is by keeping track of the way you feel when you sleep a certain amount of time. If you feel great when you get seven hours of sleep, but feel terrible after getting nine, then you probably require the amount you're getting when you wake up feeling refreshed and ready to go.

Do sleep requirements change as we age? Some experts say we require less sleep as we age. Once again I believe there is a personal physiological difference between many of us. Something that I have definitely noticed since turning fifty is that I cannot afford to miss sleep and expect to function as well as I may have when I was younger. I do best with eight or even nine hours of sleep per night.

Increasing one's daily activities has an effect comparable to taking a sleeping pill, according to researchers at the 2003 Annual Meeting of the American College of Sports Medicine.[21] In fact, exercise may

---

[21] Cox, A. (2006, June 20). Exercise: Key to good sex, good sleep. CNN. Accessed via www.cnn.com.

actually have more long-term benefits, says Shawn D. Youngstedt, Ph.D., assistant professor in the department of Exercise Science in the Arnold School of Public Health at the University of South Carolina, in Columbia. Sleeping pills can actually make insomnia worse, he says, since symptoms can worsen when patients stop taking the medications. Exercise is a safer and more effective alternative, says Dr. Youngstedt.

The National Sleep Foundation reports that exercise, especially in the afternoon hours, reduces the time it takes to fall asleep and leads to a deeper, undisturbed slumber. In a National Sleep Foundation annual poll, older adults who report more active lifestyles, such as exercise and volunteer activity, sleep seven to nine hours and complain less about sleep problems.[22]

Research has long shown a positive connection between exercise and sleep quality, but experts have yet to reach a consensus about the best time to strap on those sneakers and begin a fitness regimen.

Physicians generally recommend reserving the morning hours or early afternoon for workouts. However, few studies prove exercising right before bedtime has any negative effects on sleep. In fact, some studies actually indicate evening exercise can also improve sleep, says Dr. Youngstedt.

Research on women, who tend to report more sleep problems possibly due to hormone levels associated with menopause and pregnancy, indicates that women may draw greater benefits from morning exercise. For example, one study showed postmenopausal women who have trouble sleeping benefit more from moderate exercise plus stretching each morning. Only women who exercised

---

[22] Foley, D., Ancoli-Israel, S., Britz, P., & Walsh, J. (2004, May). Sleep disturbances and chronic disease in older adults: results of the National Sleep Foundation Sleep in America survey. *Journal of Psychosomatic Research.* 56(5), 497-502.

in the morning had a positive effect.[23] This is especially important to consider since women are twenty percent to fifty percent more likely to have insomnia than men.[24]

Dr. Youngstedt says physicians should stress that patients who are having trouble sleeping should find any convenient time to exercise, even if it is during the evening hours. The important thing is increasing activity levels and moving around. "Patients should exercise whenever they find it convenient," says Dr. Youngstedt, no matter what time of day.

Regardless, physicians need to stress the connection between better health and better sleep. "Evidence is so overwhelming for health benefits of exercise," Dr. Youngstedt says. "Better quality sleep could be just one more benefit."

If you are still having problems falling asleep and staying asleep, there are some things you can do to help yourself. Never eat right before going to bed! This can cause numerous health problems because it is hard to digest your food while lying down, and the food is more likely to be stored as fat because your need for calories are at its lowest during the resting state. If you have problems with an enlarged prostate gland then you shouldn't drink any fluids two hours prior to going to bed. Also refer to the supplement list for things that can help with this condition.

Reading in bed until you become sleepy can help you relax and get your mind off your daily affairs. You can then put your book down and get a good night's sleep. Sex is also a good way to become relaxed before going to sleep. This may sound like a contradiction to what I said about not exercising before bedtime, but sex is the

---

[23] Tworoger, S.S., et al. (2003, Nov. 1). Effect of a yearlong moderate-intensity exercise and a stretching intervention on sleep quality in postmenopausal women. *Sleep*. 26(7), 830-6.

[24] No authors listed. (2006, Jan. 10). Insomnia no more. Helping yourself get a good night's sleep. *Mayo Clinic Women's Healthsource*. 10(1), 4-5.

exception to this rule, because after it is completed most people enter an extremely relaxed state.

If you've tried all of these things and your mind is still racing, you can then try some muscle tensing/relaxing techniques. You can start by tensing and relaxing your calf muscles and work your way up your body. By the time you reach your face you should be more relaxed. To accomplish this you simply flex, or squeeze each muscle, working your way up your body, for approximately ten seconds, and then relax that muscle.

After this you should do about three to five minutes of diaphragmic breathing. When you breathe in this manner you can place your hands on your midsection, and every time you inhale your stomach will get larger, and every time you exhale your stomach will get smaller.

If you are still having problems sleeping, you can try some of the supplements listed earlier. I would try 400 mg. of magnesium at bedtime as a first effort; then I would try some melatonin. If these aren't working you could try 5-HTP, valerian root, hops, or kava kava. I've noticed in my use of melatonin that it helps me get to sleep, but doesn't seem to help me to stay asleep, whereas the other herbs mentioned help me to stay asleep through the night without interruption. There are some good formulas sold in health food stores that have a combination of these supplements. These are all relatively safe with few or no side effects.

Don't stay in bed, unless you can make money in bed.
George Burns (1896-1996)

Emotional Wellbeing

If you are going through hell, keep going.
Sir Winston Churchill (1874-1965)

Beyond a shadow of doubt our emotional state will directly affect the other two aspects of our being. When we are in emotional turmoil our physical health will suffer and our spiritual state will suffer, or when we are in love (come on now you can remember that feeling you had when you were with that special person in your life) we feel great and the world looks bright and wonderful. It is easily seen how our emotions directly affect our physical and spiritual parts of ourselves.

We must also be aware that when we have a physical problem it will affect our emotional well-being. A person suffering from a painful sickness or disease will often be in a depressed state. Thus we must learn how to improve our emotional state of being in a like manner as we approach improving our physical or spiritual well-being.

I believe one of the reasons women live longer than men is because they are generally healthier emotionally than men. Why is this? It is probably due to the fact that women are better communicators and are better at sharing their feelings with other people. Men hide their emotions and are uncomfortable in sharing them. The result is often inner turmoil.

To be emotionally healthy a person should be able to express his or her feelings in an appropriate manner. This requires having intimate (being intimate does not necessarily, or usually involve sex) relations with others. Men are not good at this either. We can talk about sports, fishing, hunting, the news, work, and other non-personal things, but we do not feel comfortable talking about our feelings. If you fall into this category you could improve your emotional health by talking with a counselor, a pastor, or at the very least, read and heed the advice given in a self-help book.

Prior to becoming a naturopathic doctor I worked as a social worker. During this time I've seen how detrimental emotional instability can be to a person's health. It can lead to substance abuse problems, other addictions, or a large assortment of other problems.

After reaching fifty most people begin to realize the value of relationships, and how other people are necessary parts of our lives. If you have a person that you trust, you should be able to share your thoughts and feelings with that person and get valuable feedback. If you do not have someone to talk with, you should begin to cultivate a relationship with other people. People who are socially active tend to live longer and have a more positive outlook on life.

Another important factor in our emotional health is our self-esteem, or in some cases a lack of self-esteem. Self-esteem is basically the way we view ourselves. Low self-esteem can lead to a myriad of problems such as addictions, problems with relationships, and health issues.

One of the best ways to improves one's self esteem is by improving our health and fitness level. By following the guidelines set forth in this book, you will undoubtedly improve your self esteem as a by-product of your wellness journey. Isn't that great news?

Other ways to improve self-esteem would be to learn new skills, either in a school setting or through self-learning. Joining social clubs and meeting new people will also improve your self-esteem. This can be accomplished by going to a church of your choice. This leads us to the next factor in achieving wellness.

I do want to add at this point that there are some emotional problems that will require the help of others to get through. This could be in the form of counseling, or finding nutritional deficiencies that could be causing a problem. There are many natural remedies to help fight depression, for example. In Germany and other European countries, St. John's Wort, 5-HTP, and Magnesium used in combination are recommended for treatment of depression the majority of the time, and there are other options. See your Naturopathic Practitioner for a recommendation if you suffer from this or other types of emotional problems.

I believe it is wise to try a natural alternative prior to using a pharmaceutical drug, but if you are already using a pharmaceutical drug, you must talk to your medical doctor about the possibility of switching to a natural alternative, and you should always dose down in the proper manner. Never just discontinue use of a drug without prior discussion with your doctor because it could lead to a serious problem. Another exception to the rule of trying natural remedies prior to using pharmaceutical drugs would be in any life-threatening situation.

Now that we've chased that rabbit we can continue our journey.

The greatest discovery of any generation is that a human being can alter his life by altering his attitude.
William James

Spiritual Wellbeing

The unique personality, which is the real life in me, I can not gain unless I search for the real life, the spiritual quality, in others. I am myself spiritually dead unless I reach out to the fine quality dormant in others. For it is only with the god enthroned in the innermost shrine of the other, that the god hidden in me, will consent to appear. **The Ethical Philosophy of Life, Felix Adler**

Spirituality is defined as a belief that we are connected to and dependent upon something outside ourselves, whether it is nature, each other, or simply the unknown. Religion, on the other hand, is a specific belief system that defines and explains that specific connection. By this definition, one does not need to be religious in order to be spiritual. Spirituality includes an array of beliefs such as feelings of love, compassion, empathy, gratitude and a sense of inner peace, all of which may have profound affects upon healing.

Just knowing there is someone, or something out there that is greater than ourselves gives us a reassurance that everything will ultimately be all right. When the weight of the world is on our shoulders the burden can be hard to handle, but when we believe there is a God out there who loves us and gives order to our universe, life becomes much more bearable. When troubling times come our way, and everyone will have them, we can believe that God will not put more on us than we can handle.

A little over seven years ago I lost a son in an automobile accident. It was the greatest loss I have ever experienced. When I was first notified of the tragedy I couldn't believe it was real, but as it began to sink in I became emotionally numb, and then all of the feelings of the loss set in. My salvation in this horrible crisis was my belief that my son was in a better place, one without suffering and pain. It may seem strange and foreign to many readers, but I actually had visions of my son in Heaven, and I believe God actually spoke to me and comforted me during this trying time. I speak from experience when

I tell you that having a spiritual connection to God will soften even the hardest of life's blows.

Taking time to pray and meditate will calm our spirits and give us an opportunity to commune with our God. Our spiritual life is usually the one aspect of our being that is the most neglected. We spend lots of time improving ourselves physically and emotionally, yet we have so little time to spend in spiritual endeavors. Of course I am speaking in general because there are some people who do spend lots of time developing themselves spiritually.

People across the world are gaining interest in spiritual healing. Unfortunately, the advent of modern scientific medicine brought about a clear separation between spiritual, religious and scientifically founded beliefs. With the emergence of holistic therapies, there has been a resurgence of interest in promoting spiritual and religious healing and in studying its effectiveness in a whole host of disorders.

It has been scientifically proven that patients in hospitals who are praying and have been prayed for recover faster than those who have not. When our innermost being is doing well, the other two aspects of our being seem to do better as well.

Spirituality includes a variety of characteristics such as a diminished focus on self, a feeling of love that leads to acts of compassion, and the experience of inner peace. There are various ways to tap into the benefits of spirituality. Examples include seeking love and support, engaging in private and intercessory prayer, developing faith, hope, and forgiveness, and participating in therapeutic touch. The key to deriving benefits from such spiritual therapies is to understand that everyone has power. Your health and your future health may be controlled by altering the external factors (diet, exercise, and other lifestyle habits) and your internal (emotional) worlds, but let's not forget about our spiritual being that dwells in our bodies.

Love, both giving and receiving, is a component of all religions. We most often demonstrate our love to those who surround us. Frequently this is to a spouse or family member, but love and social support can be given and received from all those who surround us. Its importance in ours lives and its affects on health have been studied even in childhood. Married couples also seem to live healthier lives.

People who receive emotional support from others are more likely to manage their physical symptoms more effectively during times of illness. People are more likely to quit smoking or eat healthier, for example, if friends and family encourage the change. Another health benefit of social support is stress reduction. Decreasing stress levels improves overall well being and decreases strain on all body systems, especially the heart and immune system.

Seventh-Day Adventists, who generally do not use alcohol, consume pork, or smoke tobacco, live an average of four years (women) to eight years (men) longer than other people in the United States.

I guess this emphasis on the spiritual is the one aspect that I neglect the most at this time in my life. It is usually a second thought when there is nothing else to do, or perhaps a Sunday morning exercise that many of us do. The times I've spent developing myself spiritually were probably some of the most peaceful times in my life. These were the times where I knew that ultimately everything would always work out.

So how does a person go about developing his or her spiritual aspect? I thought you'd never ask! It takes the same discipline that it takes to get to the gym or do any exercise program. Making time for prayer, doing nice things for others and expressing love and compassion requires a concerted effort on our part. We have to set some time aside, make an appointment with God, and endeavor to converse with Him. Will we always get answers to our thoughts and prayers? I'm not sure. The reason I say this is because I believe we often get answers that we do not like and dismiss them as non-answers. Once again I have to remind you that this is a journey, not a destination. In some respects this is a journey where we feel as though we are walking alone, but it doesn't have to be. Take someone's hand and take them on this journey with you, and during those difficult times allow your Maker to travel with you and allow Him to carry you through the tough times.

Things to Avoid if You Really Want to Remain Healthy

Smoking is definitely something to avoid if you truly want to achieve a state of health and, or fitness. That includes the direct smoke from your choice to smoke and the second hand smoke from others. I like to tell people that they had better be pretty tough if they want to smoke, because they are in for a life with more sickness, disease, pain, and suffering than a non-smoker.

Among the many problems associated with smoking are: various types of cancer (lung, mouth, tongue, throat, and possibly kidney), emphysema, heart disease, hoarseness, smokers cough, and chronic bronchitis. An average smoker dies about eight years sooner than a non-smoker. The major cause of this decrease in life expectancy is accelerated heart disease. The second major cause of this decrease is lung cancer. Ninety percent of lung cancer is attributed to smoking. Another problem caused by smoking is the odor of the smoker. You smell like an ashtray; your hair smells like an ashtray and your clothing smell like that also. In most cases the smoker doesn't even realize they smell that way. Many people have given up this nasty habit, and this is good news, because any time one person can accomplish something that means others can too!

It is quite interesting to note how most people realize this information about smoking to be true, but they feel as though it will not happen to them. It reminds me of the time I was driving home from work and I noticed a large amount of smoke in the air. My first thought was that there was a fire in my neighborhood. As I got closer I then thought that the fire was fairly close to my apartment, and as I got closer I realized that it was my apartment, but the thought had never crossed my mind that it was my apartment in the beginning. My point here is that we often time think we are immune to the obvious consequences of risk factors in our lives. Smoking will cause harm to your body! Just stop smoking! Cold turkey, totally abstaining from cigarettes has been shown to be the most effective way to quit. Please do it for your sake as well as those who you care about!

Excessive drinking of alcoholic beverages should be avoided. Many people argue about what excessive drinking really is? It is usually said that alcohol is a problem to a person when they cannot go without it for a prolonged period of time, or when they do drink they have other problems that arise due to the drinking (such as relationship problems, work related problems or health related problems). In my opinion alcohol is treated as a foreign substance by the body, and that is why people have an allergic reaction to it. In fact, it is that allergic reaction that people seem to strive for. Alcohol wreaks havoc on the liver, the internal organ that must detoxify your body. It lowers inhibitions giving us the excuse to do things without thinking about the consequences for what we are doing. The majority of crimes committed in this country are committed while under the influence of drugs or alcohol.

I know you have heard about the antioxidants in wine; with this in mind, I will say that a glass of wine with a meal will probably not hurt you, but there are many other better ways to get your antioxidants! If you need help unwinding after a tough day try some exercise, or if that is more than you want to do at the time try some herbal tea with relaxation properties (i.e. valerian, hops, chamomile, ginger, and others). It is impossible to drink in excess and be healthy and fit.

If you are unsure about ways to stop drinking, go to an Alcoholics' Anonymous meeting, and the people there will be more than happy to help you in any way they can. You can find listings in the local newspaper or phone directory.

Unnecessary, overused, and abused prescription drugs all lead to sickness and disease. Adverse reactions to drugs constitute one of the most serious and least talked about health problems in the United States. A study done in 1994 estimated that, among patients in hospitals alone, non-error, legally administered drugs caused about one hundred and six thousand fatalities and more than two million serious adverse reactions per year. If these statistics were factored in to the ranking of leading causes of death it would rank fifth in this country.[25]   So, as you can see prescription drugs are extremely dangerous, even when taken in clinical settings at the prescribed dosage. Do not fall into the trap of watching advertisements about prescription drugs that list all of the symptoms a person might have that would benefit from these drugs, and then start to manifest these very symptoms or have a greater degree of these symptoms. These are psychosomatic reactions to these ads.

Due to this type of advertising doctors feel pressured to give prescription drugs to their patients when asked about them. Only take prescription drugs after you have tried natural remedies first, and then give your body a chance to heal itself. The exception to this rule would be when you are in a life threatening situation.

One of the most abused prescription drugs on the market today is hydrocodone. Hydrocodone abuse has been escalating over the last decade. Hydrocodone addiction is a growing crisis in the United States. While illegal drugs like cocaine, marijuana, meth-amphetamine, and heroin remain in the headlines, many individuals may be surprised to know that hydrocodone addiction could lurk right behind them as one of the most widely-abused drugs of addiction. In fact, the Federal Drug Enforcement Administration believes hydrocodone may be the most abused prescription drug in the country. Nationwide its use has quadrupled in the last ten years, while emergency room visits attributed to hydrocodone abuse soared five hundred percent.

Hydrocodone is a narcotic that can produce a calm, euphoric state similar to heroin or morphine, and despite such important and obvious benefits in pain relief, evidence is pointing to chronic addiction. Pure hydrocodone is a Schedule II substance, closely controlled with restricted use, but very few prescription drugs are pure hydrocodone. Instead, small amounts of hydrocodone are mixed with other non-narcotic ingredients to create medicines like

---

[25] Ottoboni, Alice & Ottoboni, Fred, (2002) The Modern Nutritional Diseases and how to prevent them, Vincente Books Inc.

Vicodin and Lortab. This means they can be classified under Schedule III with fewer restrictions on their use and distribution.

Vicodin, Lortab, and more than two hundred other products that contain hydrocodone are regulated by state and federal law, but they are not controlled as closely as other powerful painkillers. The lack of regulation makes them vulnerable to widespread abuse and addiction through forged prescriptions, theft, over-prescription, and "doctor shopping" (finding those doctors that are prone to writing prescriptions upon request). Hydrocodone pills have been sold for two dollars to ten dollars per tablet and twenty dollars to forty dollars per eight ounce bottle on the street.

Subject to individual tolerance, many medical experts believe dependence or addiction can occur within one to four weeks at higher doses of Hydrocodone. Published reports of high profile movie stars, TV personalities and professional athletes who are recovering from Hydrocodone addiction are grim testimonies to its debilitating effects.

Hydrocodone is structurally related to codeine and is approximately equal in strength to morphine in producing opiate-like effects. The first report that hydrocodone produced a noticeable euphoria and symptoms of addiction were published in 1923; the first report of hydrocodone addiction in the U.S. was published in 1961.

Every age group has been affected by the relative ease of hydrocodone availability and the perceived safety of these products by professionals. Sometimes seen as a "white-collar" addiction, hydrocodone abuse has increased among all ethnic and economic groups. The most likely hydrocodone abuser is a twenty to forty year old, white female who uses the drug because she is dependent or trying to commit suicide. However, hydrocodone-related deaths have been reported from every age group.

101

Other prescription drugs that are commonly abused are pain relieving drugs, mood enhancing drugs, diet pills, performance enhancing drugs, and sleeping aids.

So what does this have to do with health and fitness? You would be shocked to find out who these pharmaceutical drug abusers are. It is likely that you know quite a few of them, but have no idea about their addiction. They work real jobs, go to church on Sundays, workout in the fitness center, and appear to be normal in every other way. It is even likely that some of our readers have or have had this problem. Hydrocodone and many of these other drugs are extremely hard on the liver. Anyone who abuses these drugs should get help and stop immediately before it ruins your life and the life of your loved ones! Try to rebuild your liver by eating right, exercising regularly, and take liver enhancing products like milk thistle on a regular basis.

As a general rule I personally believe that prescription drugs should be used as a last resort, after you have tried less harmful natural products and making changes to your lifestyle. An exception to this rule would be in any life threatening situation where you do not have time to wait for a natural product to work. I've stated this numerous times in this book because I want this concept to sink in!

Ladies, avoid the use of *Synthetic Hormone Replacement Therapy*! In a study performed by the Women's Health Initiative (WHI) about the effects of PremPro (Premarin: equine estrogen) plus Provera (a synthetic progestin) involving 16,000 women aged fifty to seventy-nine, it showed unequivocally why you should avoid this type of treatment for peri-menopause, menopause, or post menopause stages of life. Among these women studied there was a twenty-nine percent higher risk of breast cancer, a twenty-six percent higher risk of heart disease, and a forty-one percent higher risk of stroke. Other complaints from these women were weight gain, fatigue, depression, irritability, headaches, insomnia, bloating, low thyroid, low libido, gallbladder disease, and blood clots as a result of their HRT.[26]

Rather than using a synthetic hormone replacement therapy you should consider using a bio-identical hormone replacement therapy, eating a balanced diet without excessive calories, eliminate the use of refined carbohydrates, eat meat in moderation only, and exercise regularly.

Bio-identical or natural hormones are exact duplicates of what the human body creates, and synthetic hormones are not natural to the body and will be handled in a slightly different manner. Some of the popular synthetic hormones that should be avoided are: Progestins, Provera, Premarin, and PremPro.[27]

If you are taking one of these you owe it to yourself to get and read one of Dr. John R. Lee's books about menopause or hormonal balancing.

One of my arch enemies is *white sugar*. This substance should be avoided at all costs! It is one of the most detrimental substances that we can put into our bodies. It causes our liver to produce cholesterol that goes into our bloodstreams and it causes our pancreas to produce large amounts of insulin that can eventually wear out the cell receptors and cause us to acquire type II diabetes, and it will also cause other hormones to become out of balance. I have, and will, continually mention the ill affects if this substance throughout this book. I cannot overemphasize the dangers of white sugar products. Look at white sugar as if you are looking at Darth Veda, Attila the Hun, the Black Plague, or Osama Bin Laden! Become a militant white sugar hater and you will be healthier for it.

---

[26] John R. Lee, MD; Virginia Hopkins,2004, What Your Doctor May Not Tell You About Menopause, Warner Books.
[27] John R. Lee, MD; Virginia Hopkins, 2006, Dr. John Lee's Hormone Balance Made Simple, Warner Books.

White sugar has many disguises. Some of various names for sugar you will find in the list of ingredients are: glucose, sucrose, maltose, dextrose, corn syrup, syrup, corn sweetener, juice concentrate, and natural sweeteners. Some of the foods to avoid are: pies, cakes, candy, donuts, cookies, many desserts, ice cream, sweet rolls, carbonated drinks such as coca cola, etc., and fruit drinks. If you insist on eating these types of foods then learn how to make them yourself using unrefined products for the ingredients.

Other arch enemies are *white flour and white rice* because they too are rapidly turned into glucose in like manner to white sugar products, and they have the same detrimental affects to the body.

Tanning, whether it is accomplished outdoors or with the use of a tanning bed, should be also avoided, or accomplished with extreme caution.

When the body is exposed to ultraviolet radiation (UVA rays), cells called melanocytes are stimulated to produce melanin, the brown pigment responsible for the tan. As a result of tanning a greater amount of melanin is produced to protect the skin from further damage from the sun. Darker people have more melanin in their body than do lighter skinned people.

Nobody is totally immune from getting skin cancer, and in fact, some people are more susceptible to lasting skin damage depending on their skin type. Dermatologists have identified six skin types ranging from Type I, those with the fairest skin who always burn, to Type VI, skin that is deeply pigmented and never burns.

Those with Type I and II skin should always avoid prolonged periods in the sun. Those with more natural protection from the sun (Type V and VI) are at less of a risk from the dangers of tanning, but should still never neglect to protect themselves from future sun damage.

Not everyone has the time to lie out religiously at the beach to achieve a bronzed body. Since the 1980s, women started to utilize **tanning beds** to solve this problem, only to create more dangers of tanning in turn. Tanning beds emit more UVA rays in a shorter period of time than the does the sun.

While UVA rays may not burn like UVB rays, they penetrate the skin deeper, putting you at greater risk for premature aging and skin cancer. Tanning beds can also damage your eye sight and immune system, and if not properly sanitized, can be a haven for bacteria.

Skin cancer doesn't just happen to people in their forties and fifties. People as young as twenty have been diagnosed with skin cancer. Skin cancer is the number one most preventable cancer in the U.S., yet the most common. The deadliest form of skin cancer is melanoma, which if diagnosed and treated early enough can almost always be curable.

The two most common types of skin cancer are basal cell carcinoma, which grows slowly, and squamous cell carcinoma, which usually stays in the epidermis but can metastasize or spread.

To achieve the golden look minus the wrinkles and chance of skin cancer later, try tanning lotions or spray-on tans, like the Mystic Tan, which is increasingly available at local tanning salons. Tanning lotions contain the ingredient dihydroxyacetone, or DHA, which oxidizes on the skin's outermost layer, creating the look of a tan. I cannot attest to their safety because they are fairly new and no research has been done that indicates any major problems from their use, except some allergic reactions.

The results from a sunless tan can last anywhere between several days to two weeks. Tanning lotions are cheaper than spray-on tans and can easily give you the same results. To avoid unsightly streaks, exfoliate with a loofah prior to application to wipe away any dead skin cells.

Tanning Myths

A tan is healthy and protects you from sunburn. No tan from the sun is healthy. It is simply a visible sign that you have damaged your skin.

Getting a tan helps clear up acne. There's no concrete evidence to support this statement. Tanning can actually irritate the skin and if you are using certain prescription acne treatments, staying out of the sun or artificial light is strongly recommended.

The body needs Vitamin D, and tanning is a way of obtaining it. Vitamin D is indeed an essential vitamin that the skin can manufacture as a result of sun exposure, but just one hour of daily sun exposure is enough to meet the RDA for this nutrient. Everyday exposure to the sun and some foods provide adequate amounts of Vitamin D for the body. If appealing to your health doesn't strike a cord with you, think about how the wrinkles and leathery appearance might look twenty years down the road. Sun-kissed skin does look great, but you can safely achieve the same results with a sunless tan. Invest in keeping your skin beautiful and healthy, away from the sun, and avoid the dangers of tanning.

Public health experts and medical professionals are continuing to warn people about the dangers of ultraviolet (UV) radiation from the sun, tanning beds, and sun lamps. Two types of ultraviolet radiation are Ultraviolet-A (UVA) and Ultraviolet-B (UVB). UVB has long been associated with sunburn while UVA has been recognized as a deeper penetrating radiation.

Although it's been known for some time that too much UV radiation can be harmful, new information may now make these warnings even more important. Some scientists have suggested recently that there may be an association between UVA radiation and malignant melanoma, the most serious type of skin cancer.

UV radiation from the sun, tanning beds, or from sun lamps may cause skin cancer. While skin cancer has been associated with sunburn, moderate tanning may also produce the same effect. UV radiation can also have a damaging effect on the immune system and cause premature aging of the skin, giving it a wrinkled, leathery appearance.

People sometimes associate a suntan with good health and vitality. In fact, just a small amount of sunlight is needed for the body to manufacture vitamin D. It doesn't take much sunlight to make all the vitamin D you can use -- certainly far less than it takes to get a suntan! I recommend people get about twenty to thirty minutes of non-peak hour sun a day.

Yes. The number of skin cancer cases has been rising over the years, and experts say that this is due to increasing exposure to UV radiation from the sun, tanning beds, and sun lamps. More than one million new skin cancer cases are likely to be diagnosed in the U.S. this year.

Malignant melanoma, now with a suspected link to UVA exposure, is often fatal, if not detected early. The number of cases of melanoma is rising in the U.S., with an estimated 38,300 cases and 7,300 deaths anticipated this year.

Skin aging and cancer are delayed effects that don't usually show up for many years after the exposure. People who choose to tan are greatly increasing their risk of developing skin cancer. This is especially true if tanning occurs over a period of years, because damage to the skin accumulates. Unlike skin cancer, premature aging of the skin will occur in everyone who is repeatedly exposed to the sun over a long time, although the damage may be less apparent and take longer to show up in people with darker skin.

People with skin types I and II are at greatest risk. Which skin type are you?

Type	According to Skin Type
I	Always burns; never tans; sensitive ("Celtic")
II	Burns easily; tans minimally
III	Burns moderately; tans gradually to light brown (Average Caucasian)
IV	Burns minimally; always tans well to moderately brown (Olive Skin)
V	Rarely burns; tans profusely to dark (Brown Skin)
VI	Never burns; deeply pigmented, not sensitive (Black Skin)

Avoid eating in fast food restaurants because they serve overly processed foods, and they have added chemicals that may or may not be listed in their ingredients that are available for the public to view. It was recently noted that these restaurants were using large amounts of trans-fats in their foods. Some fast food restaurants are beginning to eliminate the trans-fats from their ingredients, but the majority still uses them. In general fast food restaurants serve foods that are calorie laden and nutrient depleted.

Avoid the handling of toxic materials, such as those found in pesticides, insecticides, and many types of glue, cleaning solutions, industrial solvents, and other known toxins. If you work with or around a toxin you should get a Hair Mineral Tissue Analysis on a regular basis (every three to six months) to check for heavy metal deposits. You can use various types of chelation therapy to remove toxic metals from your body.

One of the methods used is intravenous chelation therapy with EDTA. It is very effective, but should be performed by a licensed practitioner. This form of chelation may cause the recipient to feel sick, when eliminating the toxins from the body, due to the rapid action of chelation. Another form of chelation therapy is performed by ingesting a variety of minerals that will bind with a heavy metal and eliminate it from the body in a slower fashion. Rebounding on a mini trampoline, performed on a regular basis, has also been found to be effective in eliminating toxins from the body.

As stated earlier it is important to avoid getting toxins in your body in the first place. Some heavy metals may accumulate in the body due to everyday living in an industrialized society. It is probably a good idea for everyone to get a Hair Tissue Analysis at least once every few years to see if chelation therapy is necessary.

Avoid over-watching television when you could be doing something more productive. If you don't want to look like a couch potato, then don't behave like a couch potato!

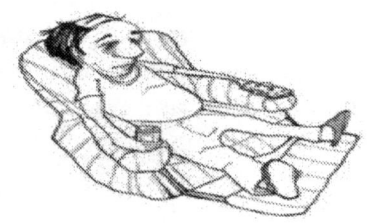

Attaining Fitness

Winners never quit and quitters never win!
Dr. Steve Fisher

General Fitness Guidelines

I don't believe one grows older. I think that what happens early on in life is that at a certain age one stands still and stagnates.
T. S. Eliot

A good fitness program will work on the various facets of fitness: cardiovascular, strength, and flexibility. I've seen many people over the years who look great, but forget to work on their most important muscle, the heart. It's like having a car with a great body design and a flimsy four-cylinder engine to run it. It looks like a race car, but doesn't run like one! I recommend everyone should find a way that suits their needs and circumstances, to train in each of the three facets of fitness on a regular basis.

Depending on your goals you will decide how often to do each per week. If you are trying to trim down and lose some weight, cardio-vascular and strength training will take up the largest part of your training time. If I were to break it down by percentages, that routine would be approximately forty percent cardio training; forty percent strength training, and the remaining twenty percent flexibility training. On the other hand, if you are trying to gain weight you would change those percentages to look like this: sixty percent strength training; twenty percent cardio training, and twenty percent flexibility training. Later I'll get more specific on how to make a routine that will give you the most benefit from your efforts.

Remember it is always better to be safe than sorry. What I mean by this is that you should begin all fitness endeavors slowly, and gradually increase the difficulty of what you are doing. A common mistake made by people over fifty is that they get out and do more than they should have. Unfortunately we do not always know we

110

are doing this when we first start. It can debilitate us the next day or even a couple of days later. Leaving us unable to continue with our program, we may just call it quits. We are on a journey, not in a race! Take your time, and add a little at a time, and before you know it you'll be working out with the twenty year olds.

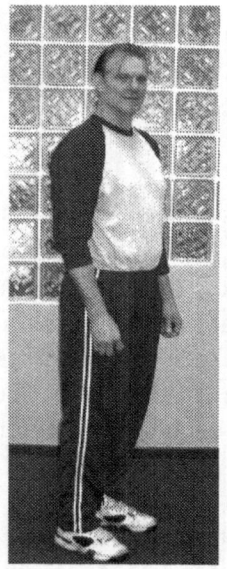

Joe M. is a fifty-three year young health and fitness enthusiast. He believes that eating healthy foods five to six times per day is the most important factor in his present state of health. Breakfast is usually oatmeal or another high fiber cereal with added protein, walnuts, and fruit. His midmorning snack contains fruit, nuts, or soy chips. Lunch is leftovers from his previous dinner and contains vegetables, lean meat, a sweet potato or brown rice. This also is what he eats for dinner, and his mid afternoon snack is similar to his other snack.

He consumes no pharmaceutical drugs or alcohol and he takes a number of supplements. They are a multi vitamin/mineral, protein, ZMA, glucosamine w/chondroitan, omega 3-6-9, vitamin B, vitamin D, and glutamine.

Joe's workouts consist of a minimum of three vigorous weight training sessions per week. For stress management Joe prays regularly and meditates on the word of God.

In the past Joe was addicted to drugs, smoked and has undergone two rotator cuff shoulder surgeries. He is truly an over comer and has used health and fitness ideals and a strong belief in God to achieve his high degree of fitness today!

Cardiovascular Training

Cardiovascular training can take on many shapes and forms. This type of training is designed to exercise the heart, lungs and systems that support these important organs. The normal heart is a strong, muscular pump a little larger than a fist. It pumps blood continuously through the circulatory system. Each day the average heart "beats" (expands and contracts) one hundred thousand times and pumps about two thousand gallons of blood. In a seventy year lifetime, an average human heart beats more than two and a half billion times. Thus for the person who will live one hundred and twenty years, our hearts will beat approximately four and a quarter billion times. Our hearts are truly miraculous organs.

The circulatory system is the network of elastic tubes that carries blood throughout the body. It includes the heart, lungs, arteries, arterioles (small arteries), and capillaries (very tiny blood vessels). These blood vessels carry oxygen and nutrient rich blood to all parts of the body. The circulatory system also includes venules (small veins) and veins. These are the blood vessels that carry oxygen and nutrient depleted blood back to the heart and lungs. If all these vessels were laid end-to-end, they'd extend about sixty thousand miles. That's enough to encircle the earth more than twice.

The circulating blood brings oxygen and nutrients to all the body's organs and tissues, including the heart itself. It also picks up waste products from the body's cells. These waste products are removed as they're filtered through the kidneys, liver and lungs. So you can see how important our cardiovascular system is to our overall health and well being. Exercise is a necessary component of cardiovascular health! So, let's take a look at ways to achieve this.

A general rule for achieving a cardiovascular effect through exercise would be to get your heartbeat to a point where you are within a certain range of heartbeats per minute. The formula for this is 220 minus your age X 60% - 80%. Let's say you are fifty years young. The formula would then look like this: $220 - 50 \times .60$ to $.80 = 102$ to 136 beats per minute. Thus a fifty year old person would endeavor to keep their heart beating 102 to 136 times per minute. The lower number being the minimal beats per minute can be used to achieve the cardiovascular effect desired and the upper number being the maximum number of beats per minute. In the beginning it is important to stay on the low end until to your body adapts to doing this type of work.

The way we accomplish this is by working large muscle groups for a certain period of time (usually twenty minutes or more). Some of the best exercises for achieving this are walking outdoors or on a treadmill (outdoors being your first choice when possible for any of the exercises mentioned), biking; swimming, rebounding on a mini trampoline, jogging (if your joints can stand the impact), rowing on a lake or on a machine, and a large variety of cardio machines you can find in a fitness center.

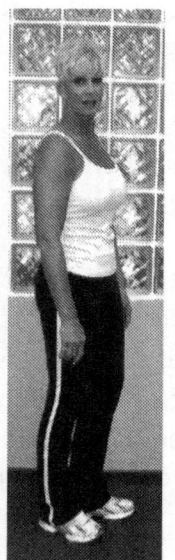

Connie W. is a fifty year young cosmetologist who looks and functions like a woman in her thirties. She attributes her present state of health and fitness to staying active through work and play. She enjoys doing yardwork, housework, cooking, working as a hair stylist, and working out regularly.

Her workouts consist of cardio training four times per week and weight training different body-parts on a rotating basis throughout the week. Some of Connie's cardio consists of walking a minimum of three miles, or walking on a treadmill for twenty minutes.

Connie enjoys eating grilled and sautéed foods, pasta, rice, steamed vegetables and salads. She admits to drinking cokes. There are no pharmaceutical drugs used on a regular basis; nor does she smoke. Connie does enjoy some wine with dinner occasionally.

113

Her supplements usage is as follows: Black Cohosh with soy isoflavones, calcium, vitamin E, B-6, and B-12; selenium, and chromium.

For stress reduction Connie feels as though doing yardwork and working out help her the most. She keeps her mind active by reading motivational books, and spiritual books.

Connie believes that people should live to ninety-five years and she doesn't expect to see a decline in her health until her eighties, but doesn't expect to see a decline in her fitness levels ever!

During the past year Connie has been faced with numerous physical problems. During this time she had an accident that injured her mouth, and was diagnosed with a malignant cancer. After undergoing two surgeries approximately six months ago, she had to lay-off from her training for a short period of time, but has overcome these health and fitness obstacles because of her outstanding level of fitness.

Connie is a wonderful example of how a person can greatly benefit from his or her effort of building and maintaining a high level of health and fitness.

Walking

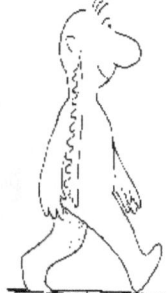

Walking is a man's best medicine.
Hippocrates

In my opinion, which was shared by Hippocrates, walking is the most beneficial exercise with the lowest risk for injury that a person could perform. Walking an extra twenty minutes per day can burn enough calories to take off approximately seven pounds of body weight per year. Longer, moderately paced walks done for about forty minutes at your lower end target heart rate (heart beating at two hundred and twenty minus your age times 60% - 65%) are best for losing weight, while faster paced walks done for twenty to twenty-five minutes are the rate of 75% - 80% of the formula are best for conditioning your heart and lungs.

Walking has so many benefits aside from the obvious ones. It helps to control your appetite, relieves stress, slows aging, reduces levels of cholesterol, lowers blood pressure, helps control diabetes, reduces the risk of colorectal, prostate and breast cancer, aids in the rehabilitation from heart attack and stroke, promotes intestinal regularity, promotes restful sleep, reduces stiffness in joints, relieves most cases of backache, promotes healthier skin due to increased circulation, improves mental alertness and intellectual creativity, elevates mood and reduces depression, increases sexual vigor, and helps to control addictions to nicotine, caffeine and other drugs. Wow! That's a lot of benefits from such a simple exercise.

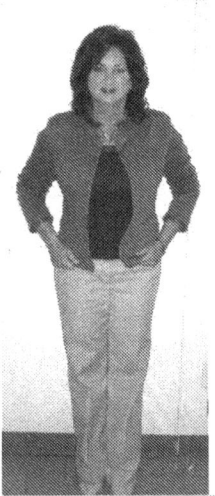

Sann T. is a probation officer who looks ten to fifteen years younger than her chronological age. She exercises consistently, walking three to four times per week, doing floor exercises, stretching, and light weight training. Her diet is healthy in that she eats fruits, vegetables, and protein dishes on a daily basis. There are no pharmaceutical drugs or tobacco products taken regularly; although she does enjoy drinking wine one or two times per week. She takes a small number of supplements, being a Multi-Vitamin/Mineral and a B-Complex tablet daily.

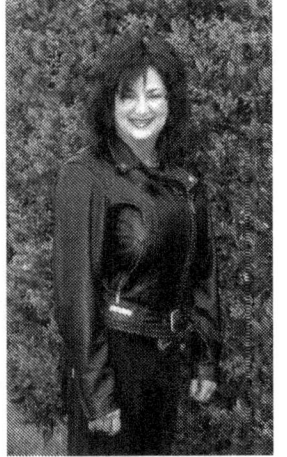

Sann takes time for relaxation and fun. She enjoys riding her motorcycle, going on group trips, and enjoys the company of others. Her attitude is generally upbeat and she almost always has a smile on her face.

I really enjoy walking outdoors and looking at the scenery. You can even see interesting things on the ground when walking. I've incorporated walking into my exercise routine for a number of reasons. I walk to and from the fitness center that I exercise at four times per week. It gets me to and from the gym without using gas; thus saving money and also saving the atmosphere from additional carbon dioxide emissions. It is also great for time management in my situation.

It is important to get the most benefit from your walk, so let's go over the proper ways to walk for fitness.

Five Points of Correct Walking

- Move at a steady pace. Feel your heart rate increase to a comfortable level. Check your pulse rate to see if you are hitting your target heart pace. The easiest way to check your pulse is to find the carotid artery on your neck and count the number of beats in six seconds and just add a zero to that number and you have your beats per minute.
- Hold your head high, keep your back straight, and tuck in your stomach. Move your feet in a straight line while moving your arms in rhythm to your steps.
- Walk by landing on your heel. Roll forward and push off from the balls of your feet.
- Take easy, comfortable strides. Do not over reach your natural walking stride.
- Breathe deeply. If you are walking briskly, you will likely find that breathing through the mouth works best.

Another consideration when walking is to choose the correct clothing for the weather you are about to face. When it is cool outside it is a good idea to dress in layers of clothing in case you become hot and need to remove something, or there is a chance of rain be prepared for that also. Be careful in extreme heat and humidity, because exercising in it can be counter productive. Only you know how hot it has to get to be considered extreme for you, and remember the higher the humidity the harder it becomes to breathe and cool down.

Be aware of your surroundings when walking. Women should walk in well lit and safe neighborhoods. You may want to carry some pepper spray with you in case you encounter a potentially dangerous dog or human. Also watch out for road hazards. Some streets have pot holes and can be dangerous. If you listen to music while you walk, be sure it is not so loud that you will not be able to hear the sound of motor vehicle traffic, or other sounds that could alert you to danger.

I realize this may sound like a lot of things to consider, but the rewards of walking in fresh air are truly amazing and worthwhile. You may also want to consider walking on a treadmill. This would give you many of the same benefits as walking outdoors without having to face any of the obstacles.

Biking

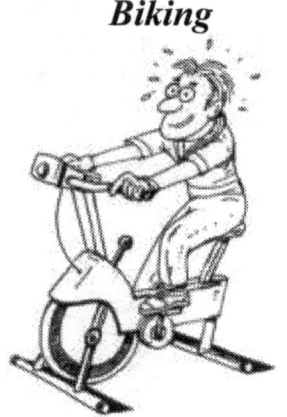

Growing old is no more than a bad habit which a busy person has no time to form.
Andre Maurois

Riding a bike would be my second choice for cardiovascular exercise, but you must live in an area that is biker friendly. Not all cities have a place for bikes to ride, and they have to share the road with other vehicles. This can be dangerous at times. I've had times when drivers of cars or trucks would try to see how close they could get to my bike without hitting me. Those events will take all the fun out of a bike ride. The seats on bikes can also be a problem for some people. I cannot understand why they can't make those seats user-friendlier. It is never comfortable to have the front part of a bike seat up your rear end. They can also cause prostate problems for some men. I have recently seen wider bike seats that you may want to consider.

The benefits of cycling are that it works the heart better than walking without pounding on a hard surface; a person could ride almost anywhere and use this form of exercise to get from one place to another, and in doing so a person would be lowering his or her overall carbon dioxide emissions (that they would have emitted if traveling by automobile).

If you live in a city that has a lined area for bikes to travel on I would recommend this as both a form of exercise and a mode of transportation. Before purchasing a bike, be sure to try a few out, and get one that best suits your needs and budget. It could be a worthwhile investment that would last for many years.

Other ways to bike would be on an upright or recumbent stationery bike. An upright bike looks similar to the one you would ride outdoors, but does not have a back wheel, and does not require any balance on your part. A recumbent bike is one where you are sitting behind the front wheel with your legs in a forward position.

You can purchase these types of bikes or go to a fitness center to use a variety of bikes that they would have. This would allow you to bike in any weather without concerns of traffic. The benefits are almost identical to what you would achieve riding outdoors, but not as intense of a workout could be achieved, and the only sites you will see are those located around the area where the bike is located.

Swimming

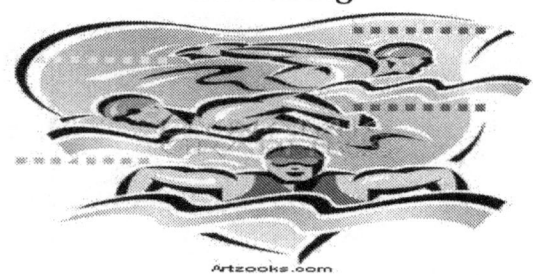

Artzooks.com

Obstacles are those frightful things you see when you take your eyes off your goal.
Henry Ford (1863-1947)

Swimming is a great form of exercise if you have access to a pool or a body of water. It is also necessary to know how to swim to use this as an exercise form. If all of those prerequisites exist, then you can exercise without putting much stress on your joints. The exception to this being easier on the joints would be the rotator cuff, which is located on your shoulder area. Swimmers do have a tendency to get overuse syndrome problems. Overuse syndrome problems occur when joints are used over and over in high repetition types of work or exercise.

The benefits of swimming are it improves posture, flexibility, endurance, strength, and balance; it stimulates circulation, creates muscle tone, promotes deep breathing, and helps to control and maintain a healthy weight. A good workout can burn three hundred and fifty calories per hour! It does not put any pressure on your joints, so it is better than many other exercise regimes such as running. It is a great stress reducer and it increases your energy level.

Swimming can serve as a cross-training element to your regular workouts. Before a land workout, you can use the pool for a warm-up session. Swimming, with increasing effort to gradually increase your heart rate and stimulate your muscle activity, is easily accomplished in the water. After a land workout, swimming a few laps can help you cool-down, move blood through your muscles to help them recover, and help you relax as you glide through the water.

Swimming does burn calories at a rate of about three calories a mile, per pound of bodyweight. If you weigh 150 lbs. and it takes you thirty minutes to swim one mile (1,760 yards or 1,600 meters), then you will be using about nine hundred calories in one hour. However, many swimmers do not swim that quickly, and many cannot swim for that distance or duration.

Spending time in a group workout, whether water aerobics or a master's swim practice, is a great social outlet. Exchanging stories, challenging each other, and sharing in the hard work make swimming with others a rewarding experience.

There are other psychological benefits to swimming, if you allow it to occur. Relax and swim with a very low effort. Let your mind wander, focusing on nothing but the rhythm of your stroke. This form of meditation can help you gain a feeling of well-being, leaving your water session refreshed and ready to go on with the rest of your day. Many swimmers find an indirect benefit from swimming. They develop life skills such as sportsmanship, time-management, self-discipline, goal-setting, and an increased sense of self-worth through their participation in the sport.

Jogging

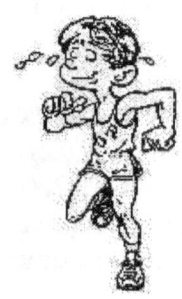

Old age isn't so bad when you consider the alternatives.
Cato

Jogging is an excellent form of exercise, but does impact your joints drastically. If you have been a jogger for a while, and have no detrimental effects from it, then by all means continue to incorporate it into your exercise regime. The benefits of jogging are many, but I feel as though the risk for the over fifty group outweigh these benefits!

Although I am biased against jogging, I still want to be fair and let you, the reader, decide for yourself on your course of action.

Like walking, jogging is an aerobic exercise that is easier to learn than some of the other activities such as swimming or cycling. Jogging burns more calories than you would if you were walking for the same amount of time. It is also easy to do while away from your home on business or a vacation. While packing for a business trip just throw those sneakers in the suitcase and you'll be ready to go.

So what is the difference between jogging and running? There is no one definition for both, but basically jogging is performed at a slower pace than running. Running a mile in less than nine minutes is considered running, while running slower than a nine minute mile is considered jogging.

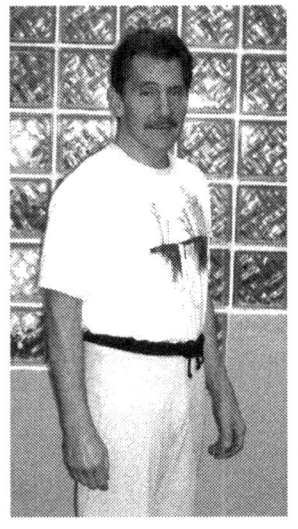

Ronny V. works in the insurance industry. He attributes his high degree of health and fitness to "consistent attention to exercise, nutrition, and supplementation." He has never smoked, drinks very little alcohol, and takes no prescribed medications.

As a child Ronny says he was overweight, and by the age of ten he became interested in fitness and was determined to lose that excess weight. Two fitness obstacles that he has overcome were a torn right biceps tendon and then nine years later, a torn left biceps tendon. Each injury required that he lay off from training for four months. This was discouraging for him because he is an extremely disciplined and dedicated individual.

Ronny expects people to live past a hundred, and never expects his health or fitness levels to decline. He works out diligently, running seven days per week and weight training five days per week. He watches his diet closely, taking in no sugar, trans-fats, fried foods, diet drinks, or artificial sweeteners. The mainstay of his diet is whole grains, fruits, and vegetables.

Ronny's supplementation regime is extensive: multi- vitamin/mineral, trace minerals, liquid herbs, noni juice, hyolauronic acid, chlorophyll, fish oil, enzymes, probiotics, and EDTA on a daily basis. He also does a total body cleanse twice per year.

Ronny, at fifty-nine, is in better shape than most twenty year olds! I worked out in the same gym as Ronny about fifteen years ago, and he has maintained a high level of fitness throughout his lifetime. Most people would assume that he is about forty years old.

If you are determined to start jogging you should do it as safely as possible. Start out by walking with short periods of jogging. Two minutes of walking followed by one minute of jogging is a good starting place. Slowly decrease the amount of walking until you can jog continuously for twenty minutes.

Find a good running shoe that is made for your foot and body structure. Go to a store where the sales people are runners. Look for good cushioning, plenty of toe room, and a snug fit at the heel.

Make sure you warm-up properly to avoid injuries and follow your workout with a cool down period consisting of walking and then stretching.

Try to maintain proper form when jogging by keep your eyes focused ahead of you with your head lifted; avoid looking at the ground since it can cause problems with your upper body posture and lead to upper back and neck pain. Keep your shoulders relaxed and chest out and open and do not lean forward. Do not over arch your back and stick your rear end out either, as this can cause back and hip pain, and keep your arms close to your body. Swing arms forward and back, but do not swing them across the body and don't clench your fists.

Once again I want to reiterate the fact that jogging is beneficial and can add to one's health and fitness levels, but it can lead to injuries if one is not extremely careful in the way you approach this exercise. So, if you decide to jog do so with care and caution!

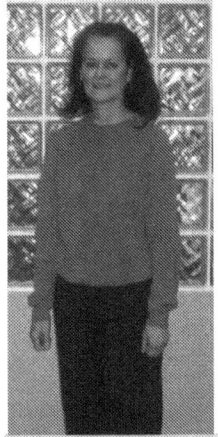

Ava S. is a fifty-three year young women who has run almost everyday for the past twenty-eight years. Her good health and fitness are attributed to her daily running, being careful about the choices of food she eats, and never smoking or drinking.

She eats several light meals each day, and drinks mostly water. Her protein is mainly derived from poultry and fish. Her supplements include a daily multi vitamin and extra vitamin E and vitamin C. More than fifteen years ago Ava was diagnosed with a heart defect and

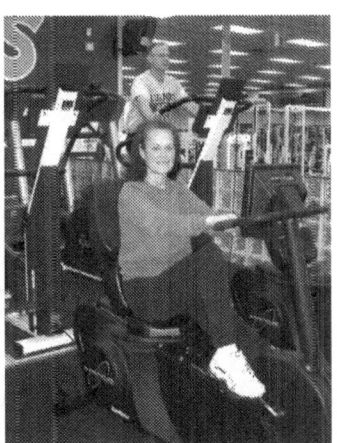

a pacemaker was placed in her body. This in itself would deter most people from continuing to train on a regular basis, but it didn't in Ava's case. She continued to train until this day and expects to do so for many years in the future.

It is due to this dedication and perseverance that Ava looks and functions years younger than her chronological age.

Rebounding

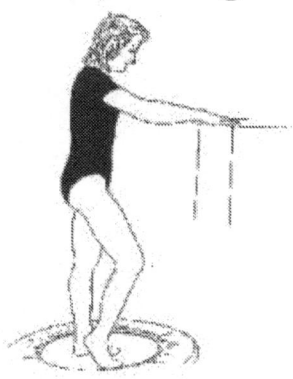

Rebound exercise on the mini trampoline is yet another form of cardiovascular training. Because it moves all parts of the body at once we can also call it a cellular exercise. When we think about the bodily functions, we know that the heart is the pump for the blood, but the lymphatic system does not have a pump. It is only moved by physical activities, and rebounding is the perfect activity because it gets everything moving at once. As a cellular exercise rebounding not only gets the juices flowing, but it also helps to remove toxins and then deliver and absorb nutrients at the cellular level where it can be converted into energy.

As an exercise it is superior to many others because it not only uses gravity but also two other forces, acceleration and deceleration. At the top of the bounce you experience weightlessness, and at the bottom your weight doubles pulling you into the center of the mini trampoline.

As a therapy it is as beneficial as massage or reflexology, since the whole body is involved; it is truly a cellular exercise.

The main benefits of rebounding are as a cellular strengthener. It has detoxification effects which help rid the body of toxic metals and accumulations of unneeded minerals by circulating the lymphatic fluids, thus it is considered a natural form of chelation therapy. It strengthens the immune system by increasing the white blood count, increases oxygen delivery and blood flow, promotes mind-body unity, and is easy on the hips, knees and ankles. It actually works on all four facets of fitness: strength, aerobic capability, flexibility and endurance.

You can start rebounding for five minutes and work your way up to thirty minutes, or forty minutes, if you have the time. It is a good idea to get a high quality rebounding mini trampoline that gives a gentle bounce, and because you do not want to experience a fall from a cheap, inferior product. Although rebounding is mentioned last in this chapter, it is probably the most beneficial cardiovascular exercise of them all, with the least amount of risk of injury to joints.

As mentioned previously, most fitness centers have a broad range of machines that can make your cardiovascular workout fun, challenging, and interesting by switching machines on a regular basis. Try them all on different days, and you will find the ones you like most and this will be helpful in sticking with a routine.

Strength Training

A winner never stops trying.
Tom Landry, Ex Head Coach of the Dallas Cowboys

When we think of strength training the first thought that comes to mind is lifting heavy weights. This is why many people shy away from strength training. They feel as though they are not as strong as others and feel discouraged before they give it a chance. In actuality strength training should be called progressive resistance training. This gives us a better picture about what we will be doing. Progressive resistance simply means that we are gradually increasing the resistance that will be placed on our muscular and skeletal systems.

According to a study done by the CDC (Center for Disease Control), adults who regularly engage in strength training are less likely to experience loss of muscle mass, functional decline, and fall related injuries than those who do not. Due to the health benefits, federal officials have made a national objective, for the year 2010, to increase the proportion of adults who strength train to thirty percent (currently estimated at twenty percent of our adult population). Researchers say it is never too late to start. Inactive adults who start strength training achieve rapid gains within a few months.[28]

This should be encouraging for anyone who has been relatively inactive and wants to attain health and fitness after they have turned fifty. Now we will continue on our journey and learn more about strength training.

Let's go over some basic terminology. Your routine is the schedule that you will try to adhere to. It tells you what days to do what exercises, and tells you what exercises you will be doing. A repetition is doing an exercise one time completely. When performing

---

[28] http://aolsvc.health.webmd.aol.com/content/atricle/125/115956.

most exercises you will perform six repetitions to twenty repetitions of a given exercise. A set is when you have done the given number of repetitions of that exercise. Let's say you've done eight repetitions; then rested for one minute, and then did another eight repetitions. That would be a total of two sets of eight repetitions.

The speed of the movement is also an important element of each exercise. A reasonable training pace is one to two seconds for the lifting (concentric) portion of the exercise and three to four seconds for the lowering (eccentric) portion of the move. Fast, jerky movements should be avoided. They place undue stress on the muscle and connective tissue at the beginning of the movement, substantially increasing the likelihood of an injury. Fast lifting also cheats you out of some of the strength benefits. When lifting at a fast pace, momentum (not the muscle) is doing a good deal of the work.

Full range of motion is an important component of proper form. Each exercise should be taken through the complete range of joint movement in a slow controlled manner, with emphasis placed on the completely contracted position. If a weight is so heavy that you have to jerk, bounce or swing to get it to the top of the movement, it's too heavy to be using. Your form will be compromised if you train in this manner.

Full-range of motion movements contract and strengthen the muscle you're working (the prime mover) and stretch the opposing (antagonist) muscle. This contributes to both muscle strength and joint flexibility. An example of this would be when you are flexing your biceps (front portion of upper arm) muscle and you are stretching the triceps (back portion of upper arm). The opposite of this also is true. When you are flexing your triceps you will be stretching your biceps.

Progressive resistance is the key to any well designed strength program. This means that as your muscles adapt to a given exercise, you need to gradually increase the resistance or increase the number of repetitions to promote further gains. You should start out with a weight that allows you to do at least eight repetitions of a particular exercise. Once you can complete twelve repetitions with that weight, you increase the weight by about five percent. Now, you're doing eight repetitions with the slightly heavier weight. Once you've worked up to twelve repetitions with the heavier weight, you increase it by another five percent (or no more than ten percent) and go back to doing eight repetitions. The idea is to keep alternately increasing repetitions and resistance, so that you continue to see results.

Increases in muscle size and strength do not occur while you're training, they occur during the rest period between workouts. This is when your muscles recover and rebuild, gradually becoming bigger and stronger. The recovery process takes at least forty-eight hours. For this reason, strength training sessions should be scheduled no more frequently than every other day. If you prefer to train more often, you should avoid hitting the same muscle group on consecutive days

Always remember we are not competing against anyone but ourselves. You do not want to put yourself in an embarrassing position as did Ben Stiller, the comedian, while doing the bench press exercise at the gym one day, Ben Stiller found himself pinned beneath a barbell, screaming for help. He was pleased to have another bodybuilder help him out. He was less pleased when that bodybuilder - a dainty woman - offered him a word of advice: "Use less weight."

The goal is do a little more each time we train. Sometimes a little more may mean one more repetition, while other times it may mean more weight, and still other times it may mean less rest between sets. Never try to lift the same as a friend or co-worker just because your ego dictates you to do so. It could injure you. You may have some days where you are just glad you made it to the gym, and making progress is not even the goal for this type of day. A lighter easier routine may be more beneficial for this day.

A good routine will work all of the major muscles of the body each week. The major muscles of the body are your frontal legs, back portion of the legs (hamstrings and calves), upper back; lower back, chest, shoulders, abdominals, biceps, and triceps. Forearms are receiving a workout every time you grasp a weight or bar, and we will not have to give them much attention because of this. The exception to this would be if you are trying to increase forearm strength for a specific sport.

There are many ways to accomplish getting a good workout. You can work your entire body three times per week alternating days (i.e. Monday, Wednesday and Friday); you can split your routine and work each body part twice per week (i.e. Monday, Thursday, and Tuesday, Friday), and even split it further to work each body part once per week (this would be done four or five days in succession). I prefer to cycle my progressive resistance training and do each of these for about four to six weeks before going to the next type of split routine.

When working on the four day split routine you could work chest, shoulders, and triceps on Monday and Thursday. Then on Tuesday and Friday you would work on your legs, back and biceps. There are numerous ways to split a routine, but this is one that is used quite often by many people.

The next type of split routine would look like this: Monday you work on chest and triceps; Tuesday you work on back and biceps; Thursday you work on legs; and Friday you work on shoulders and traps (the muscles that are just below your neck and directly above your upper back).

Some people enjoy doing full body workouts year round, and that is fine. Do what suits your needs and schedule, but do something in the way of progressive resistance training!

After doing all of these routines for four to six weeks each, you may want to take a week off, doing what I call an active layoff. While resting from the progressive resistance training you still do things like walking, biking, swimming, yoga, etc. I think it is extremely important for the after fifty group to remain active year round.

Before I go into greater details about specific exercises and the various types of equipment one can utilize, I want us to decide whether or not we will need to go to a fitness center or workout at home. Going to a fitness center doesn't always mean paying for a membership at a club. Nowadays many apartment complexes have small, but generally adequate fitness rooms.

At this point you will have to do some self-examination and be honest with yourself. Am I a self motivated individual? Do I get distracted easily? Can I stick to a scheduled routine? If you are the type of person that can make up your mind to do something and you get it done no matter what, you are probably a candidate for working out at home. I would recommend this if, and only if, this is what you choose to do because it would fit your needs and schedule. I say this because many people enjoy going to a fitness center for the social aspects of it, greater variety of equipment, others trying to accomplish similar goals, and a host of other benefits. I personally enjoy going to the gym. It is something I look forward to. Perhaps I am the exception to the rule, but it is something to consider when making that decision as to join a gym or buy home equipment.

If you choose to join a health club, you should check out a variety of them that are either close to your home or close to your workplace, or on the way to either of these. Make sure it is fairly easy to get to, or it may make it easier for you to skip workouts. After narrowing down your search by location, look at the clubs and see if they have adequate amount of equipment for the number of members they have. You can accomplish this by going to the gym at 5:30 PM on a Monday. This is when the gym is usually the busiest. If the fitness center appears to be acceptable to you, go to the next step and check out the bathrooms and other amenities for cleanliness. Nobody likes to workout in a dirty facility. Ask the staff questions and see if they are knowledgeable and courteous, and if they offer instruction on how to use the equipment. If all of these conditions exist, ask them for a free one or two week pass to try out the facility. Most fitness centers offer free passes.

Now you are ready to make an informed decision as to which gym to join. Not all gyms charge the same. Some offer corporate rates for people who work at certain places. While others offer various types of deals, do not fall for the first time visit deal that they say will not be available after today! That is just a sales trick to pressure you into joining at that moment. You can usually haggle over price and they will accept you later on with the deal first mentioned. Believe me, I know the tricks of this trade because I have owned and operated fitness centers for many years.

On the other hand, if you have decided that you would do just fine working out at your home, you will now have to purchase the equipment necessary to accomplish your goals. The first place to look for equipment is from the classified section of your newspaper or from those trade papers that are used to sell a variety of items. Now you must figure out how many square foot you have in the room you've chosen to be your exercise room, and then look for equipment that will fit in that room. Never spend a lot of money on equipment until you see if working out at home is something you still enjoy after a couple of months. Otherwise you will be one of those people placing an ad in the paper to sell your equipment at a lot lower price than you paid for it.

The key pieces of equipment to purchase in the beginning are: dumbbells (a variety of weights), a flat bench, an exercise ball, cross training shoes (I like New Balance shoes), and bring a good attitude and self motivation.

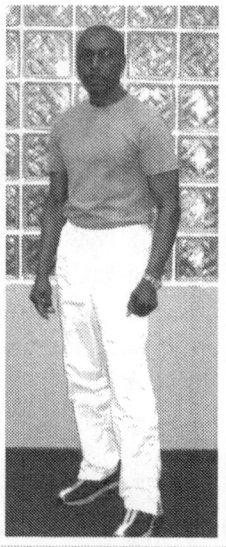

Charlie H. is sixty-eight years young and looks as though he could be in his forties. He credits blessing from God, genetics, lifestyle and daily prayer for his present state of health. His high level of fitness is due to his determination, dedication and commitment to his exercise program. He recently underwent a hernia operation and has recovered remarkably well.

Four days per week Charlie does thirty-five minutes of cardiovascular training and four days a week he performs weight training. He eats turkey, fish, chicken, vegetables, fruit, and orange juice daily. He eats nuts in moderation, and drinks approximately twenty-four ounces of water per day. He totally avoids soda and tobacco products, but drinks wine, beer or vodka in moderation on a daily basis.

To combat an allergy problem he takes an antihistamine regularly, and he supplements his diet with a multi vitamin/mineral, vitamin E and protein powder daily. He deals with stress by reflecting on Scripture and realizing that God is ultimately in control of everything.

Exercise Recommendations for the Over Fifty Group

The list of exercises below are the ones that I feel are most beneficial for the over fifty group. These exercises have the smallest risk factor for injuries and will yield the best results. You will see the terms compound movement and isolation movement next to each exercise. A compound movement is one in which you incorporate a group of muscles to perform a movement. The primary muscles used are where the exercise will be listed. An isolation movement is one in which a muscle is isolated as much as is possible.

135

This list is not inclusive. There are other exercises that may be beneficial for you to do that are not listed here. Once again the reader is encouraged to do additional research for a greater variety of weight bearing exercises. This is a great place to start.

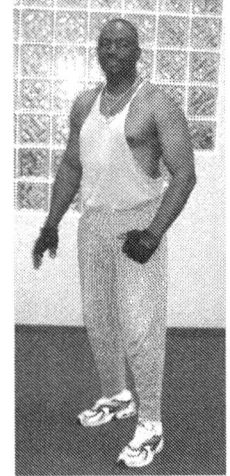

Jimmy G. has recently retired from the tire building industry and is starting on new endeavors at this time. I have personally known Jimmy for more than fifteen years and can attest to the fact that he is dedicated to health and fitness. He works out regularly and watches what he eats. His dietary regime is pretty simple, in that he eats three meals per day, includes fruits and vegetables daily, and drinks six to eight glasses of water per day. He doesn't drink alcoholic beverages, smoke, or take any pharmaceutical drugs on a regular basis.

He includes a modest amount of supplementation in daily routine. These are a multi-vitamin/mineral designed for the fifty plus group, protein, and creatine. For stress reduction Jimmy believes exercise is the key for him, and he has strong spiritual beliefs that help him concentrate on positive things in life.

While writing this book Jimmy had to undergo surgery to repair a hernia. Shortly after his surgery he was back in the gym involved in an active recovery. He should be as good as before in a few short months. When a person is in shape they can undergo surgery and get back to where they were in a lot less time than an out of shape individual.

Leg Exercises

Strong legs will serve a person well throughout one's life. They give us balance, help us lift things and travel from one place to another, and can be a beautiful and sensual part of the female body or add sex appeal to the male body.

Your legs are comprised of many muscles. The front portion above the knee is called the quadriceps. The back of your leg above the knee is the hamstring, and below your knee in the back portion are your calves. The compound movements for your legs will also work your glutes (rear end), and your lower back to some degree. You will not see barbell squats on my list because they have an extremely high risk factor for lower back and knee injuries. Perform these and all exercises as indicated previously with slow to moderate movements, never jerking in motion.

- *Compound Movements for Upper Legs:*

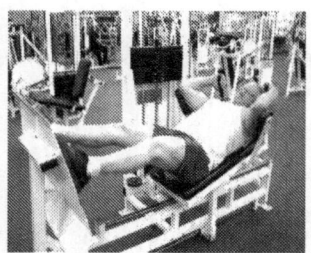
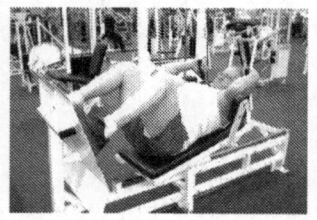

Leg Press Machine: You can do this with both legs at one time, or you can do this one leg at a time. One leg at a time is recommended for those who have had back injuries or are concerned about not getting a back injury. When using one leg at a time you will use less than half the weight and it will help to correct any strength imbalances you may have in your legs. To do this exercise you simply sit on the padded seat area and press your feet on the platform in a forward direction. You should perform three or four sets of eight to twenty repetitions.

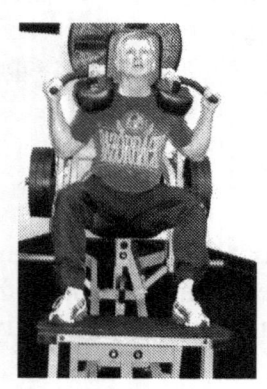

Machine Squat: When doing a machine squat make sure that the machine you are using has safety features in case you exhaust your muscles and cannot get back to the upright position. Always start off with a light weight that you can easily do until you get used to the machine you are using. After getting into the proper position under the pads you will bend your knees until they are slightly above parallel. If you feel any pain in your knees or back return to the starting position immediately and discontinue doing this exercise. After reaching the bottom position you simply return to the upright position (do not totally lock out with you knees). Start off very light and easy with this exercise because it can cause extreme muscle soreness. Perform three or four sets of eight to twenty reps once you have adapted to this exercise.

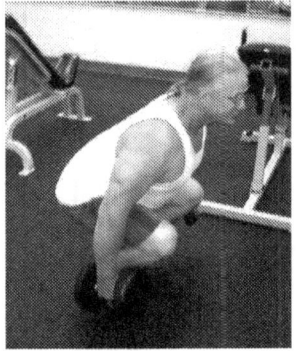

Dumbbell Squat: When doing dumbbell squats you hold two light dumbbells in your hands and bend your knees until they are slightly above parallel, and then return to the upright position. Try to stand as straight as possible without rounding your back. Always maintain proper form throughout the exercise. Perform three to four sets of eight to twenty reps.

Step-Up Squat: You will need a sturdy flat bench and a pair of dumbbells to do the step-up squat. Place the bench in front of you (the long way) and grab a pair of light dumbbells. Place one foot squarely on the bench and lift yourself up by straightening your leg. You should have both feet on the bench at this point. Now step off the bench leaving the same leg squarely on the bench and then bring the other leg to the ground. Then repeat using the 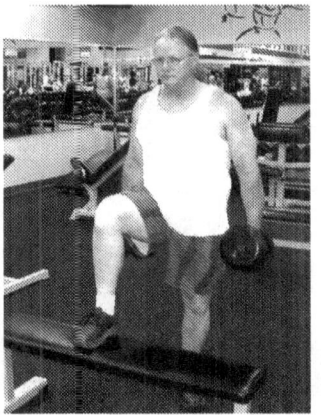 other leg. Use caution when attempting this one because it will require you to maintain your balance. Start off doing this exercise for week or so without using any weights other than your bodyweight. Perform two or three sets of six to twelve reps when you feel you are ready.

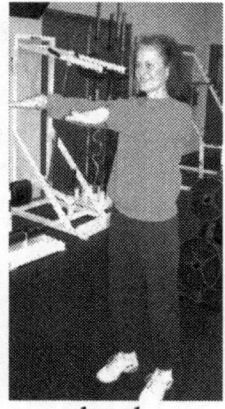
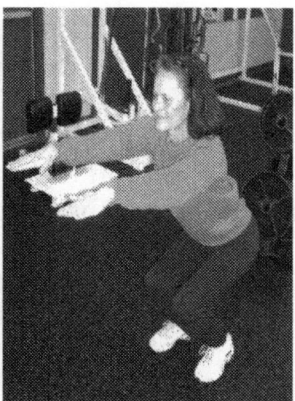

Free-Hand Squats: You will require no equipment to accomplish this basic exercise. Simply place your hands in front of you with arms outstretched, and bend at the knees until your thighs are slightly above parallel. Then stand up and you have just completed one repetition. This is a good one to do during commercial breaks while watching television. You should begin with as little as ten reps and work upward from there.

- *Isolation Movements for Quadriceps:*

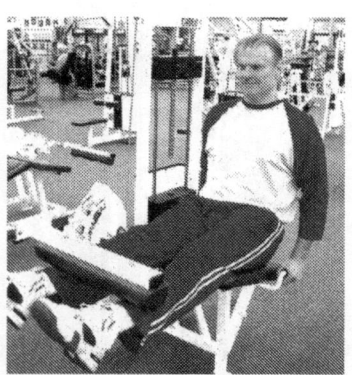

Leg Extensions: Seat yourself on the pad so that your knee is comfortably on the end of the seat and where you are not overextending your knee. Place your feet under the padded bar; straighten both legs, and hold on the top position for a second or two before lowering the padded bar. Start off light and be sure you feel no pain in the knee region when doing this. You should feel the frontal leg muscles working and possibly feel a slight burn. Perform three to four sets of eight to twenty reps.

Leg Extensions (one leg at a time): This is the same as above, but you will do one leg at a time. Keep the unused leg back behind the padded bar next to the other leg without incorporating it into your movement.

- *Isolation Movements for Hamstrings:*

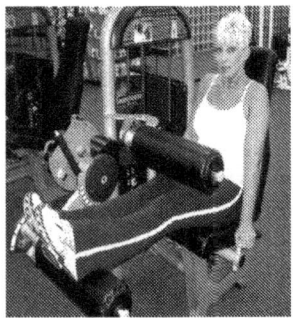

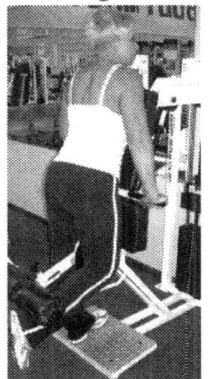

<Leg Curls (seated): While sitting on the machine you will place your feet on top of a pad and bring your heels down towards the floor. Perform three to four sets of eight to twelve reps.
Leg Curls (standing): > While standing place your feet under the pads and bring one foot up towards your rear end. Perform three to four sets of eight to twelve reps.

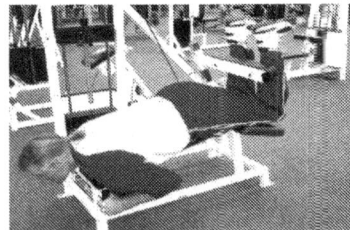

Leg Curls (lying face down): Lie face down on the machine placing your feet under the pad and bring your heels from your foot toward your rear end. Start off light and perform three to four sets of eight to twelve reps.

- *Isolation Movement for Calves:*

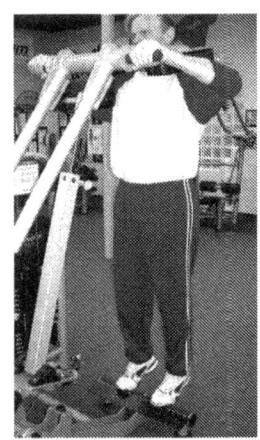

Standing Calf Raise: Position yourself with your shoulders under the pads and place your feet (the balls of your feet) on the platform. Now raise your heels as high as they will go, pause for a second or two, and then lower your heels to get a good stretch in your calves. The calves require higher repetitions because they are accustomed to a high workload from walking on them regularly. Perform three to four sets of ten to twenty reps.
The standing calf raise exercise can also be done with no weights (another one that will be good to do while watching commercials on television).

140

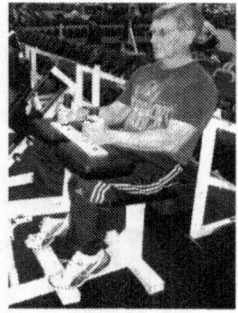

Seated Calf Raise (either one or two legs at a time): Sit on the specialized machine and place your thighs under the pad and feet on the platform. Perform this in a like manner to the standing calf raise except your knees will be bent at a ninety degree angle. Perform three to four sets of ten to twenty repetitions.

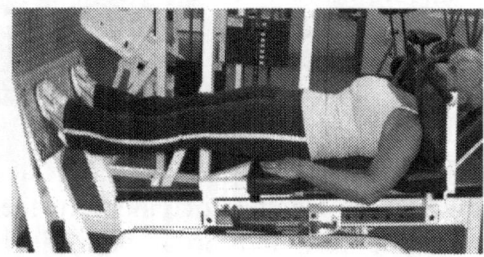

Calf Raise on Leg Press Machine (either one or two legs at a time): Sit on the padded portion of the leg press machine and place your feet on the platform. You can do this one with either straight or slightly bent knees. Perform in a like manner to the other calf raises, and do three to four sets of ten to twenty reps.

Back Exercises

Your back is also comprised of many muscles (i.e. the rhomboids, latisimus dorsi, and spinae erectors). For simplicity sake we will call them the upper back and lower back areas. Building a wide upper back can help to make a waistline look smaller, even when the waistline stays the same size. It's a sought after optical illusion that most bodybuilders incorporate to their advantage.

Once again I want the reader to know that I only list those exercises that have the least amount of risk of injury. For this reason I do not recommend anyone over fifty to perform bent-over rows, deadlifts, or good morning exercises. If you do not know what I'm talking about then do not worry about it. For those of you who may have worked out many years ago and performed these types of exercises I recommend that you forget about them as well. The benefits do not outweigh the risks of injury!

- *Compound Movements for Upper Back:*

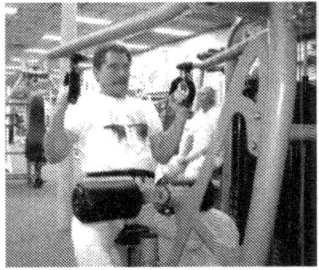

Latt Pulldowns: This requires the use of a Latt Machine. Sit on the seat and grab the overhead hanging bar (palms facing away from you) at a slightly greater than shoulder width position, then pull the bar toward your chest as you concentrate on bringing your elbows down and back, and then return the bar slowly to the overhead position. Perform three to four sets of eight to twelve repetitions.

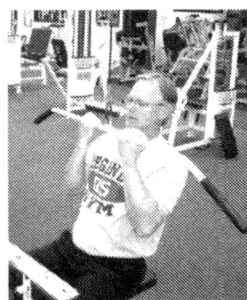

Reverse Grip Pulldowns: This is the same as the above exercise with palms facing towards you and your grip should be closer (hands approximately ten to twelve inches apart).

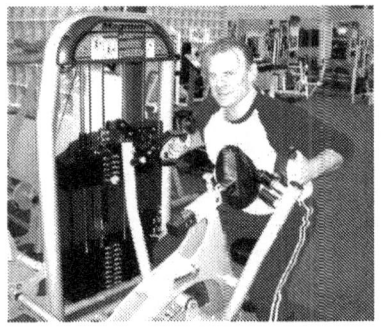

Machine Rowing: While sitting upright on the padded seat grab the handles in front of you and pull them toward your chest area. Concentrate on bringing your elbows back as far as you comfortably can. Perform three to four sets of eight to twelve repetitions.

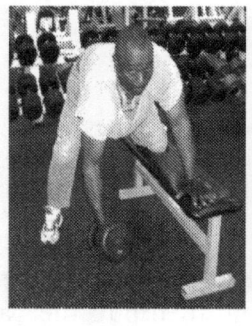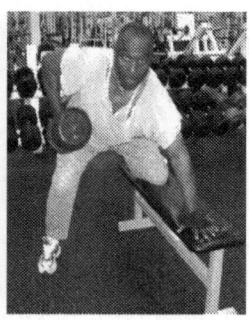

One Arm Rowing (Dumbbell): Place a dumbbell on the floor next to a flat bench, place one knee on the bench and the other leg back on the floor for balance. Now grab the dumbbell and bring it up to your outer chest area, and then slowly lower it. This exercise resembles starting a lawn mower; if you can picture that you should be able to perform this exercise. Perform three to four sets of eight to twelve repetitions.

- *Isolation Movements for Lower Back:*

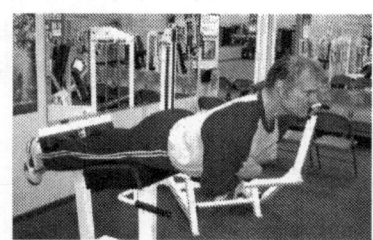

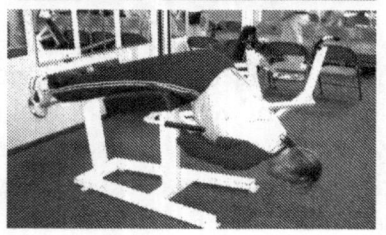

Hyperextensions: This requires the use of a specialized bench that most fitness centers have. Lie face down on the padded area with your feet under the rollers for support. Your waist should be at the end of the padded area and then raise your head, neck, and upper back as far as you comfortably can. You can do higher reps with this exercise once you are accustomed to it. Perform ten to thirty repetitions (only one set is necessary when you are doing higher reps). If you are doing ten reps per set you can do two or three sets.

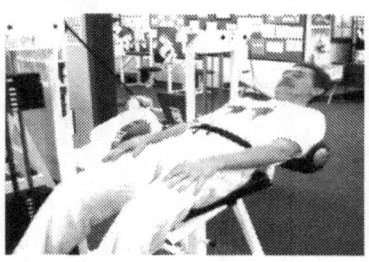

Machine Hyperextensions: Position yourself on the padded seat and the other pad on your upper back. Now lean backward as far as you can comfortably go. Each machine is

143

slightly different; thus I will not go into details about positioning. Perform two to three sets of eight to twenty repetitions. Be careful when first starting this exercise because the machine you are using may not be suited for a person of your physical height or structure; thus causing undue strain and torque on the lower back area.

Chest Exercises

Your chest is comprised of two main muscles. They are the pectoral major and pectoral minors. They are usually referred to as pecs or pectorals. Men are admired for having a large, well-shaped chest and women can enhance their breast measurement by enlarging the muscles directly beneath them. A woman's breasts are composed of predominantly fatty tissue and cannot be toned or enlarged by exercise other than the illusion created by enlarging the muscle beneath them. Because they are comprised of fatty tissue a change in diet can help to reduce their size if that is what is desired.

In recent years I've noticed that I was having more injuries to my elbows and shoulders from doing bench presses with a barbell or dumbbells, so I changed to using a variety of machines to perform these types of exercises and haven't had to deal with shoulder or elbow injuries. Some years ago I also learned, through trial and error, to never lock out (completely straighten my elbows) at the end of a movement, and this has saved my elbows from injury. If we protect our joints they will serve us well for many years to come!

- *Compound Movements for the Chest:*

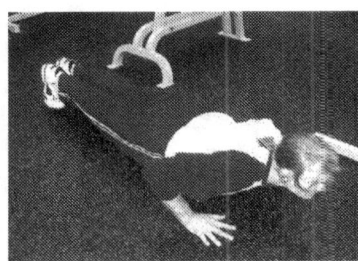 *Pushups:* No equipment is necessary to perform this exercise. Lie face down on the floor and place your hands right outside your chest area, and push your body away from the floor until your arms are almost straight (do not lock out your elbows

144

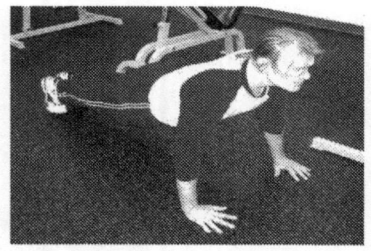

while performing this exercise). You can start out with six to eight repetitions and work upward from there. This is another one of those exercises that can be done during commercial time while watching television. If you have had problems with your shoulders or elbows use caution when performing this exercise.

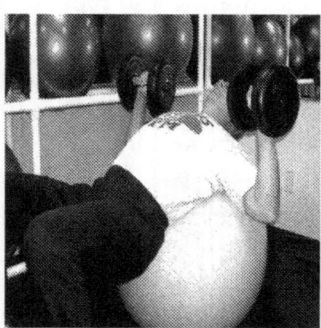 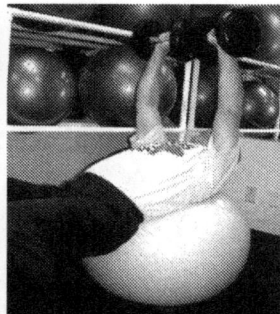

Dumbbell Bench Press on Exercise Ball: While lying with your upper back on an exercise ball you press a pair of dumbbells towards the ceiling until your elbows are extended, but not locked out. Perform eight to twelve repetitions in each set.

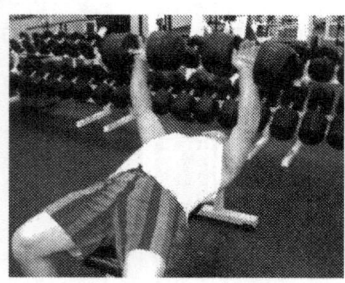

Dumbbell Bench Press: Lying on a flat bench with a dumbbell in each hand, press the weights towards the ceiling until your elbows are extended, but not locked out. Perform eight to twelve repetitions in each set.

Dumbbell Incline Press: Lying on an incline bench with a dumbbell in each hand, press the weights towards the ceiling until your elbows are extended, but not locked out. Perform eight to twelve repetitions in each set.

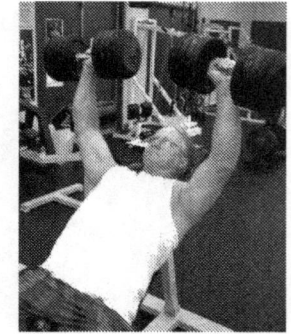

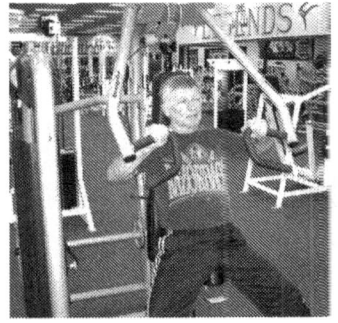

Machine Bench Press: Sitting upright on the padded seat, grab the handles and push the weights forward until your elbows are extended, but not locked out. Perform eight to twelve repetitions in each set.

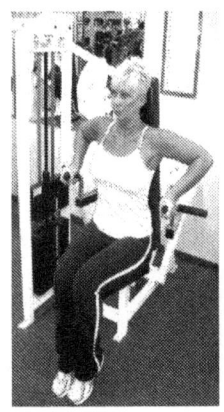 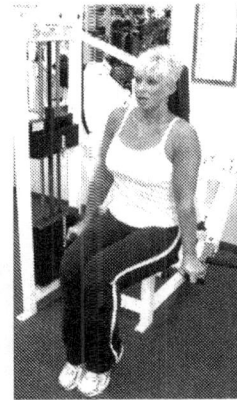

Machine Dips: While seated, grab the handles and push the weights downward until your elbows are extended, but not locked out. Perform eight to twelve repetitions in each set.

- *Isolation Movements for the Chest:*

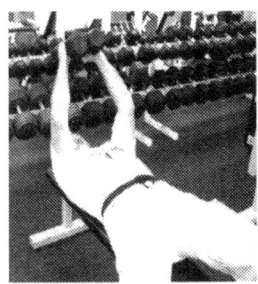 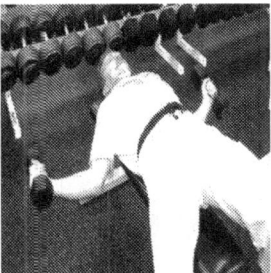

Dumbbell Flyes on Flat Bench: While lying on a flat bench, with a dumbbell in each hand, bend your elbows slightly and bring your arms downward while maintaining a constant position with your arms. It will look like you are hugging a tree when you return to the starting position. Perform eight to twelve repetitions in each set.

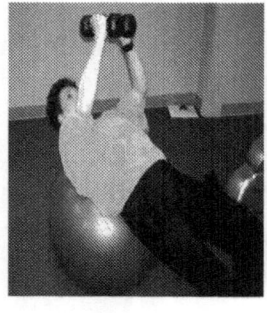 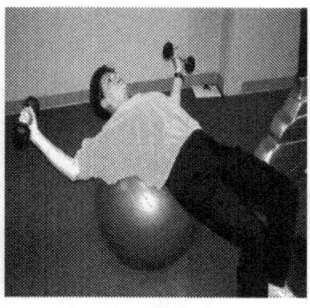

Dumbbell Flyes on Exercise Ball: While lying on an exercise ball with dumbbells in hand bend your elbows slightly and bring your arms downward while maintaining a constant position with your arms. It will look like you are hugging your spouse when you return to the starting position. Perform eight twelve repetitions in each set.

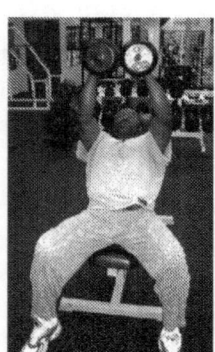 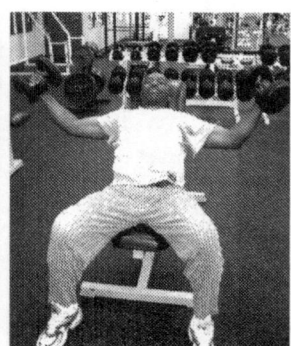

Dumbbell Flyes on Incline Bench: While lying on an incline bench with a dumbbell in each hand, bend your elbows slightly, and bring your arms downward while maintaining a constant position with your arms. It will look like you are hugging your child when you return to the starting position. Perform eight to twelve repetitions in each set.

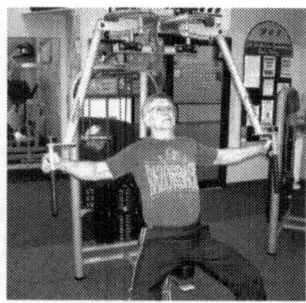 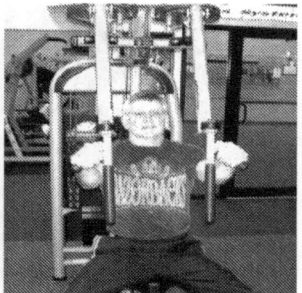

Seated Upright Machine Flyes: While seated upright grab the available handles and bring your arms forward like you are hugging a telephone pole, and then return to the starting position. Perform eight to twelve repetitions in each set.

147

Shoulder Exercises

Your shoulders consist of three heads on a muscle called the deltoid. They can help to give the body the illusion of width, thus making the waistline appear smaller. Having broad shoulders creates a desired look for both men and women because of this phenomenon. The rotator cuff joint provides movement for this muscle and is somewhat delicate in nature. We must use caution when working this area. Start out lifting light weights and you will do just fine. I will also include the trapezoid muscles in this section because it is right next to the shoulder muscles connecting your upper back to your neck.

- *Compound Movements for the Shoulders:*

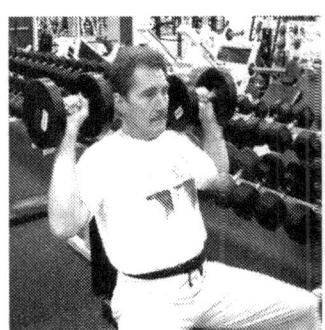 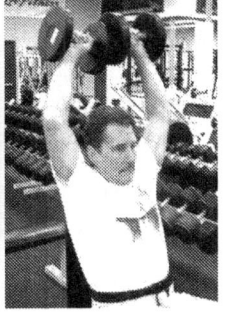

Seated Press with Dumbbells: Grab a pair of light dumbbells and sit on a bench, preferably one with a back support. Starting with your palms facing, you press the weights overhead while rotating your palms so that they are facing away from you. Do not lock out your elbows in the top position. Perform eight to twelve repetitions per set.

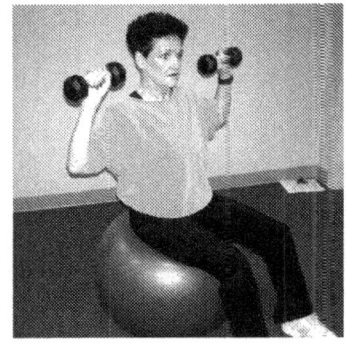

Seated Press with Dumbbells on Exercise Ball: This is the same exercise as explained above except that you will be sitting on an exercise ball while doing it. This will give you the added benefit of working your core muscle groups (midsection, front and back).

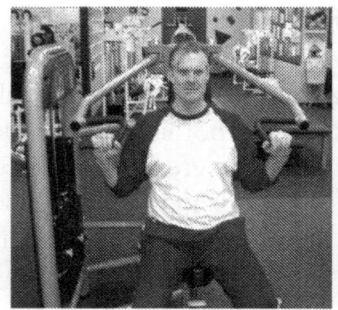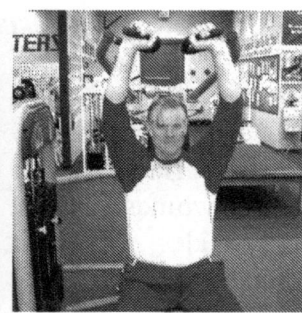

Seated Press on Machine: While seated on the padded seat grab the handles and press them upward without locking out the elbows. Perform eight to twelve repetitions each set.

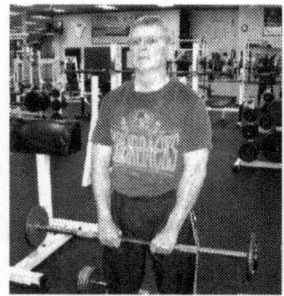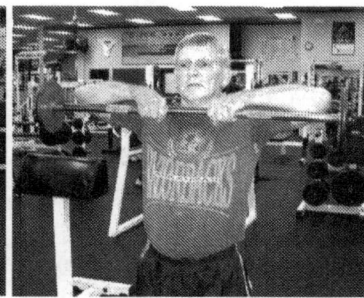

Upright Rowing: Place a barbell on a waist high rack if one is available; grab the barbell in the middle leaving approximately eight inches between your hands. Stand upright while placing one foot more forward than the other (this takes pressures off the lower back) and slowly raise the bar until it is just below your chin, then lower the bar. Perform eight to twelve repetitions per set.

- *Isolation Movements for the Shoulders:*

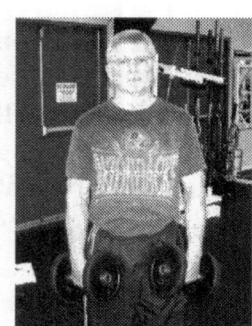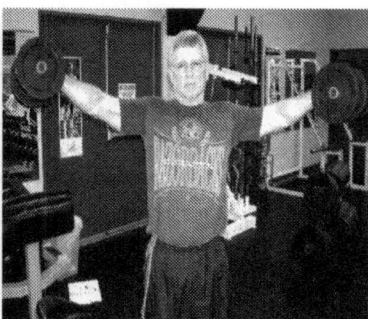

Side Lateral Raise: Grab a light pair of dumbbells and stand upright with them at your sides. Place one foot further forward than the other, and with your elbows slightly bent, bring the dumbbells upward like you are pouring water with two pitchers at one time, and then return the dumbbells to your side. Perform eight to twelve repetitions per set.

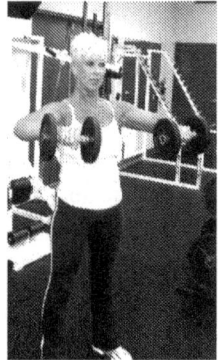

Front Lateral Raise: Grab a pair of dumbbells as listed above, but place the dumbbells in front of your thighs. Raise one dumbbell at a time, keeping your palms facing the floor, in front of your body until it reaches shoulder height, and then do the other side in like manner. This constitutes one repetition. Perform eight to twelve repetitions per set

Rear Lateral Raise: While seated on a bench, bend over until your midsection is close to your thighs. Keep your arms almost straight, but never locking the elbows, and then raise the two dumbbells towards the ceiling and return to starting position. Perform eight to twelve repetitions per set.

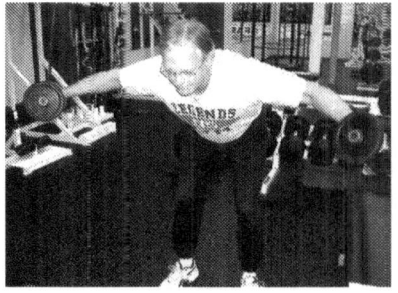

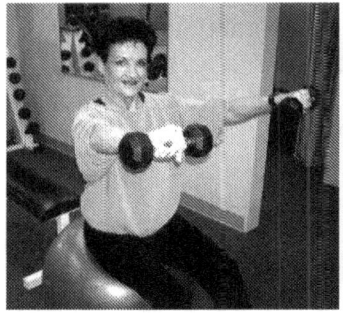 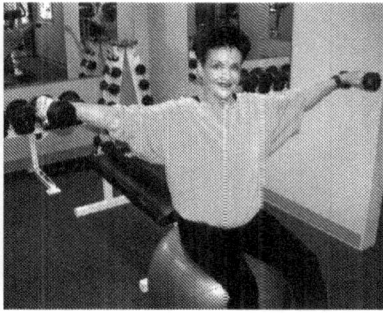

Lateral Raise on Exercise Ball: You can perform each of the three

mentioned lateral raises on an exercise ball and receive the added benefit of working your core muscles at the same time.

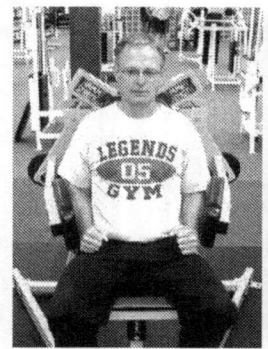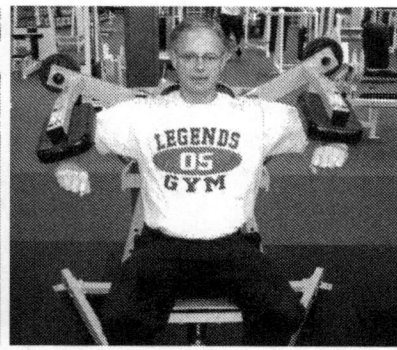

Lateral Raise Machines: You can perform the various lateral raises on specific machines that are built for each exercise. The benefits of using one of these machines can be the support you get for your lower back, and the prearranged pathway forces you to use proper body positioning.

- *Isolation Movements for the Traps:*

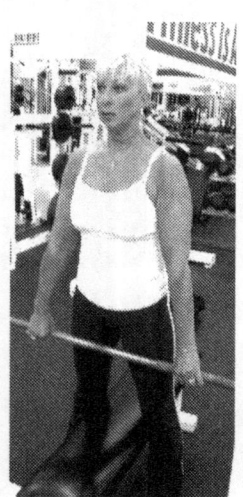

Barbell Shrugs: While in an upright position grab a barbell from a rack that is approximately two to three feet from the ground. Your palms should be facing your body and the bar will be close to your thighs. Now you will raise your shoulders toward your ears as if you are indicating that you do not know something (thus the name shrug), and then lower the bar. This is one repetition. It is a relatively easy exercise and a person could use a substantial weight while performing it, but I caution the reader to learn the proper form of this exercise before trying to lift heavier weights. Perform eight to twelve repetitions per set.

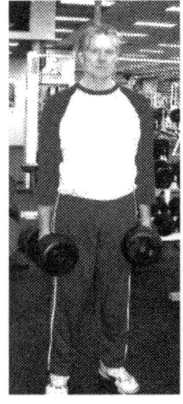 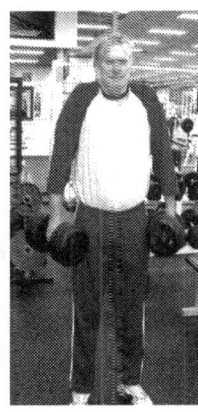

Dumbbell Shrugs: This will be performed exactly like the previous exercise, except you will grab a pair of dumbbells instead of the barbell.

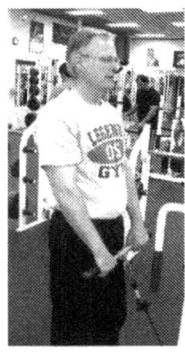 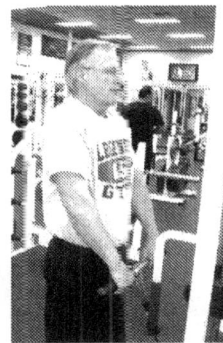

Cable Shrugs: Using a cable apparatus, attach a straight bar to the bottom portion of the cable. Grab the bar and stand upright while leaning away from the machine slightly. You will perform this exercise the same way as the previous ones.

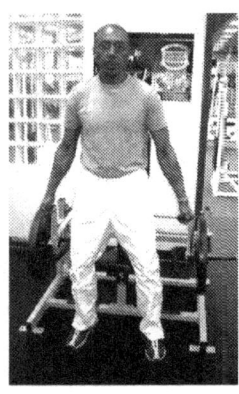

Machine Shrugs: There are machine built specifically for shrugging. Simply place the desired amount of weight on the weight holders and perform the exercise in the same manner as previously mentioned.

Triceps Exercises

Your triceps are located on the back portion of your upper arm. This area can be a problem for women in general. When the triceps lack tone they give that flabby arm appearance. So ladies, I want you to be sure to include at least one of these exercises in your program. The triceps are almost twice as big as the biceps and thus require a greater workload to get them to grow or tone. Whenever you perform a pushing compound movement (as in working the chest or shoulders) you will be working your triceps to some degree. Because of this I will only list the isolation movements for the triceps. If any of these exercises you are performing causes pain in the elbow joint, discontinue the use of that exercise and try another one.

- *Isolation Movements for the Triceps:*

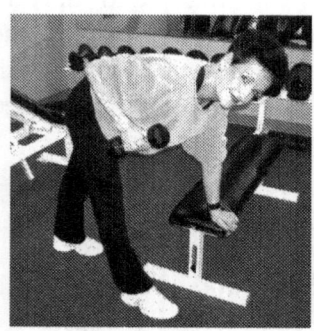 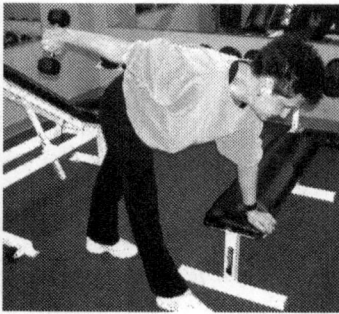

Triceps Extension: Grab a light dumbbell in one hand, and then bend over creating a ninety degree angle with your forearm and upper arm and use your free hand to brace yourself on a bench or other sturdy object. While maintaining a ninety degree angle by bending at the elbow joint, bring the dumbbell back, keeping it alongside your body, until your arm is fully extended. You will feel a tightening of the triceps muscle you are working. If you want to make this exercise even more effective, twist your hand outward after you have straightened your arm. Perform eight to twelve repetitions per set.

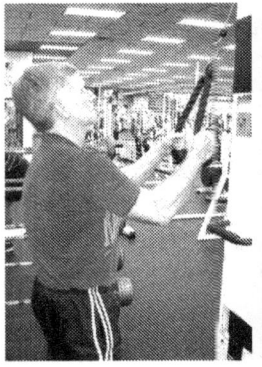 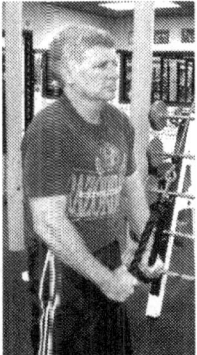

Triceps Pushdowns on Latt Machine: Grip a straight or angled bar with your hands about six inches apart, and push the bar in a downward motion, keeping your elbows at your side, until your arms are extended. It is important to keep your elbows positioned at your sides during the performance of this exercise. Perform eight to twelve repetitions per set.

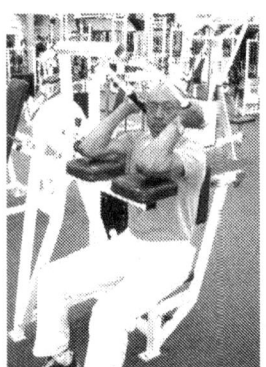 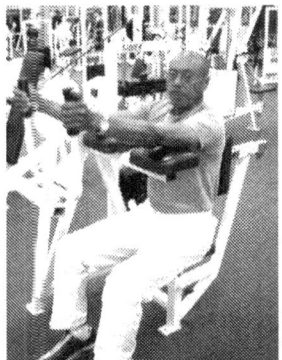

Triceps Extension on Machine: Sit upright on the padded seat and place your arms on the padded area which will be approximately shoulder height, then grab the handles and push them forward until your arms are extended. Perform eight to twelve repetitions per set.

Biceps Exercises

The biceps are located on the front portion of the upper arm. They are a very popular muscle that helps to fill out your shirtsleeve. Whenever someone says, "Let me see your muscles," people often show off their biceps in a flexed position. Having strength in your arms can make everyday tasks a lot easier. Your biceps are a small muscle group compared to others like the quadriceps, or chest muscles, so they do not require as much work to get them to grow. You use your biceps any time you perform a pulling compound movement (as in working the upper back). For this reason I will only mention the isolation movements for the biceps.

- *Isolation Movements for the Biceps:*

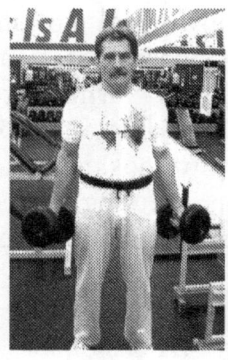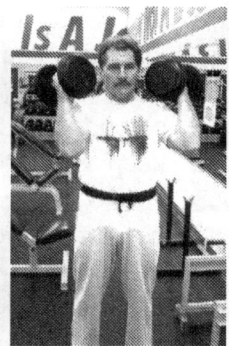

Dumbbell Curls: Grab a pair of light dumbbells with your hands facing toward your body, and stand with a shoulder width stance and one foot slightly (six to eight inches) in front of the other foot (this helps to take pressure off the lower back region), then begin to raise the dumbbells turning your hands to a palms facing away from you position, until they are at shoulder height. Then slowly lower the dumbbells while turning your hands back to the starting position (hands facing your body). Perform eight to twelve repetitions per set.

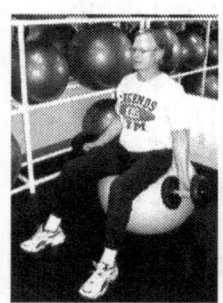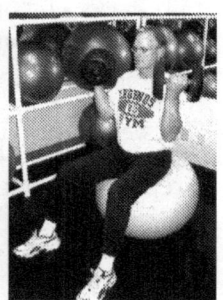

Dumbbell Curls on Exercise Ball: This is the same exercise as the one listed above, except you will be sitting on an exercise ball. This will force you to incorporate core muscles and make this a more efficient exercise. Perform eight to twelve repetitions per set.

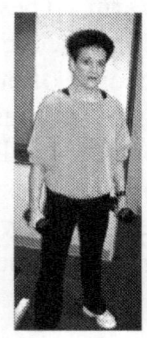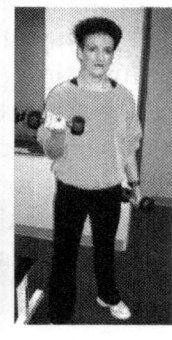

Alternate Dumbbell Curls: While standing in the same position as listed in the regular dumbbell curls you will raise just one arm at a time. One repetition is when you have curled both arms. Perform eight to twelve repetitions per set.

155

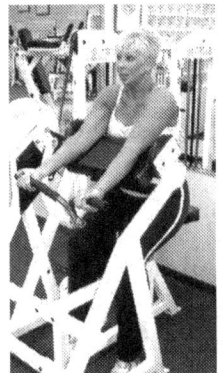 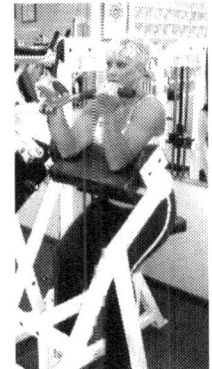

Seated Machine Curls: While sitting on the padded seat position your arms on the padded curling area and grab the handles, then curl the weights towards your chin area and slowly lower the weights. Perform eight to twelve repetitions per set.

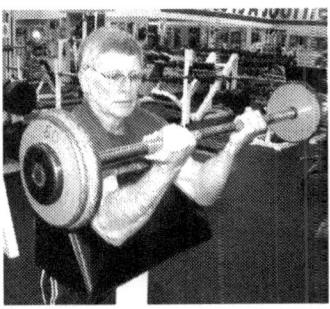 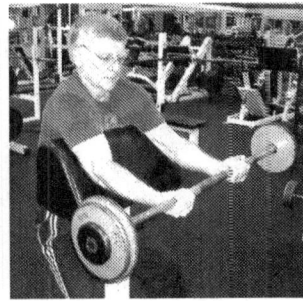

Preacher Bench Curls: Place your arms over the padded section of the preacher bench and grab a light barbell from the rack (usually in front of this bench), then curl the bar towards your chin area, and slowly lower the weight to starting position. Perform eight to twelve repetitions per set.

Abdominal Exercises

The abdominal muscles give us that flat stomach so often sought after. If we have a high degree of definition you can even see that proverbial "six pack" that men would give their right arm for. Many people foster the false assumption that you can reduce fat from your midsection by performing countless repetitions of abdominal work. This is far from the truth because you cannot spot reduce fat (unless it is done surgically) from the human body. The primary way to reduce fat from the midsection is to take in fewer calories per day from our diet than we burn each day. We can only accomplish this in a healthy manner by adjusting our workload or by modifying our diet.

With all of that said I still want the reader to know that working the abdominal muscles are still extremely important because they help us maintain our upright posture, and they keep our internal organs in their proper position. Working this area also aids the digestive process. Abdominal weakness is often associated with back pain, and if you have ever had any you know it is wise to do everything in one's power to avoid a recurrence. If any of these exercises causes you to have back pain discontinue doing that exercise immediately and find another exercise that does not hurt the injured area.

- *Isolation Movements for the Abdominals:*

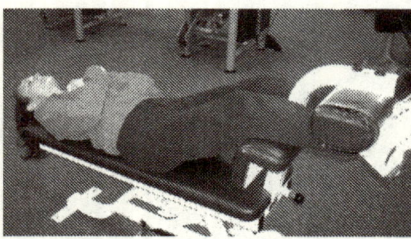
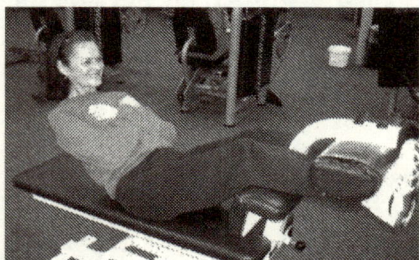

Crunches: You can perform crunches while lying on a flat bench, or on the floor. While lying on one of these, bend your knees approximately ninety degrees (leave feet on the floor or bench unless the bench is specially equipped with a place for your feet), then place your hands crossed over on your chest, and bring your head towards your knees. You will only move slightly forward making sure to leave your lower back on the floor or bench. You should feel your abdominal muscles contracting. This is a relatively easy exercise and should be done in high repetition (twenty to one hundred or more) each set.

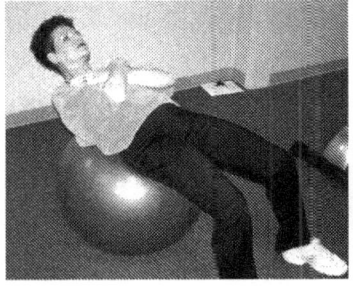 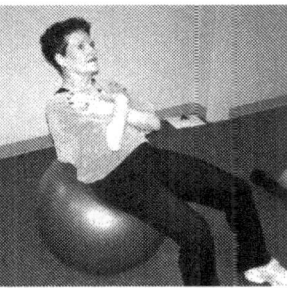

Crunches on Exercise Ball: This is performed basically the same as regular crunches except for the positioning on the ball. Your feet will remain stationery on the floor and you will sit back on the ball making sure to leave your lower back on the ball at all times. This is a little more difficult to perform than the regular crunch, but I believe it to be a more effective exercise. You should do ten to fifty repetitions of these each set.

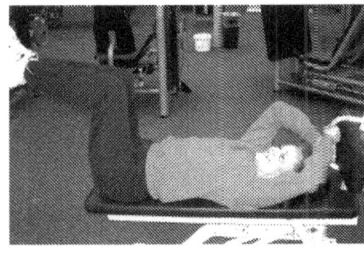

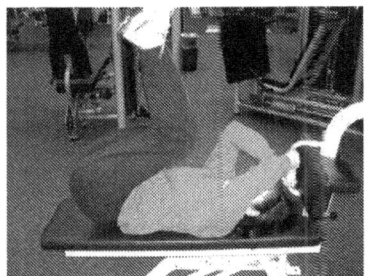

Reverse Crunches: These are done by lying down on your back; holding on to the back of a bench with your hands, raise your legs up off the bench until your lower legs are parallel to the bench (a ninety degree angle). While maintaining this position, bring your knees towards your head lifting from your midsection until your knees are about ten inches from your head. Once again your upper back will remain in contact with the bench. This is a difficult exercise to perform and should only be attempted by someone who has worked out for a year or more. Perform ten to twenty repetitions during each set.

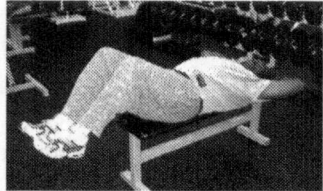

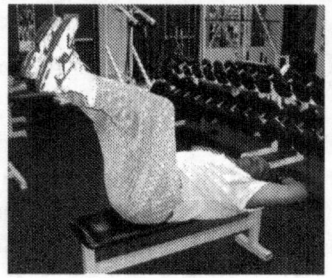

Leg Raise: While lying flat on a bench, allow your lower legs to hang over the end of the bench. With your knees slightly bent, bring your legs up to a ninety degree angle and then return them.

This is also a difficult exercise and should not be attempted by anyone who has not trained for at least six months. Perform ten to twenty reps per set.

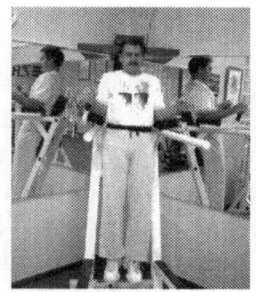

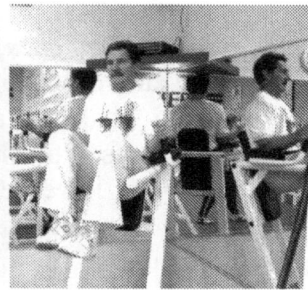

Knee Raise on Special Apparatus: This special piece of equipment will have a padded area to place your elbows and fore- arms on while gripping handles, and a padded area for your back to rest on. After you have positioned yourself on this equipment, you will bring your knees up towards your chest. This exercise can also be done on a chinning bar while in the hanging position. Perform ten to twenty repetitions per set.

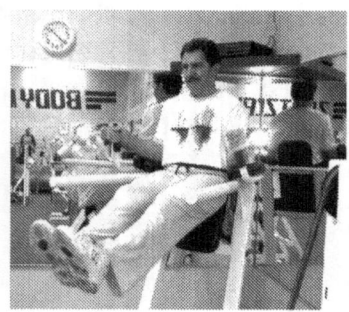

Leg Raise on Special Apparatus: Using the same piece of equipment described above, you will bend your knees slightly and raise your legs to a ninety degree angle. You can also do this exercise while hanging from a chinning bar. This is a little more difficult than the knee raise described previously. Perform eight to twenty repetitions per set.

Flexibility Training

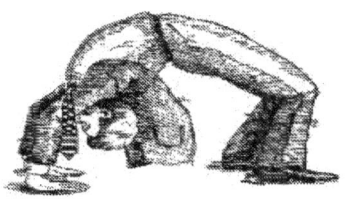

Flexibility is the forgotten segment in fitness. When ignored, it can affect your health in many ways. As you age, your muscles tighten and the range of motion in a joint can be minimized. This can put a halt to active lifestyles and even hinder day-to-day, normal motions. A regular stretching program can help lengthen your muscles and restore youthful activity. The following are some of the benefits of stretching:

- Maintain flexibility by preserving your range of motion
- Promote circulation by increasing blood and nutrients to the tissues
- Prevent injury during exercise to improve your performance and reduce your risk of injury
- You'll reduce muscle soreness and improve your posture
- You'll help reduce lower back pain
- You'll improve your coordination and help develop body awareness
- You'll enjoy your exercise more and help reduce stress
- Prepare the muscles for more vigorous activity
- Relax your mind

After a person becomes fifty years young, it becomes more important to remain flexible than it did at a younger age. Have you ever watched a baby go into all types of contortions with no effort whatsoever; and as teenagers can you remember all the things we could do without any additional efforts on our part? These benefits of youth gradually wear down through the years. We can get by with maltreatment of our bodies until we reach a certain age (and by all means I do not advocate mistreating your body) and if you are reading this book you are probably past that point now!

 A person who has tight muscles is more apt to acquire injuries due to a poorly aligned skeletal structure. Muscles left to their own devices will shorten and atrophy. This can lead to backaches, headaches, neck aches, and even knee problems. So, as you can see, flexibility should definitely be a part of your fitness regiment.

Flexibility can be achieved in a variety of ways. Working opposing muscle groups during strength training will help to some degree (i.e. working the biceps and the triceps, or working the quadriceps and the hamstrings) to maintain flexibility, but the best method to use would be to directly stretch each muscle group.

I enjoy doing yoga to maintain flexibility. It has helped my flexibility immensely. I am going to explain to you some basic forms of stretching without going into yoga at this point. Please remember that you can choose yoga movements after your strength training to achieve a high degree of flexibility. If you choose to take that route refer to the coming section on yoga.

General Stretching Guidelines

Stretching should be done in a warm environment. You should never attempt to stretch a muscle when it is cold. A simple experiment will show you why this is important. Place a rubber band in your freezer and allow it to get very cold. Now take it out and pull on it. It will probably break easily. If you take another rubber band and let it sit in the sun on a warm day or near a heater you can pull on it and it will stretch to a high degree without breaking. Your muscles are just like that rubber band! So be careful not to overstretch cold muscles.

The best time to get a good stretch and to help your muscles cool down is at the end of your workout. Many people get confused when they see athletes warming up and stretching prior to their games. The reason they do this is because they are about to perform at their maximum capacity, and without warming and stretching prior to doing this they place themselves at risk for injury.

When I stretch after my workout I do a combination of static stretching and yoga movements (many of which are quite similar). Start out stretching an area gently and gradually. Always stop at the point where the stretch gets harder or you feel discomfort in another part of your body. Hold a stretch for a given number of breaths (anywhere from ten to thirty). As you take each breath you can go deeper into the stretch you are performing.

Diaphragmic breathing is a good thing to practice while stretching. It is accomplished by breathing completely utilizing your diaphragm. To learn to do this place your hands over your stomach, and as you breathe in, allow your stomach to get larger, and as you exhale allow your stomach to get smaller. This will get air into and out of the entire lung. You will find this very important as you learn about yoga in the next chapter. This type of breathing can also be done as a stress reliever. You can do this virtually anywhere imaginable for a few minutes and it will calm your spirit.

Listed here are just a couple of stretches (this is by no means an all-inclusive list of stretches) for each muscle group:

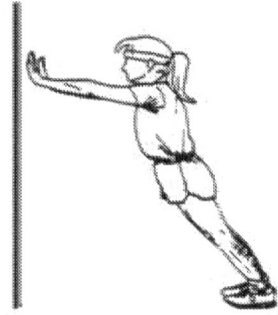

Calf Stretch on Wall: I prefer to stretch my calf muscles first. To accomplish this you can lean towards a wall with your feet about four feet from the wall keeping your heels on the ground at all times.   Hold this position for ten to thirty seconds.

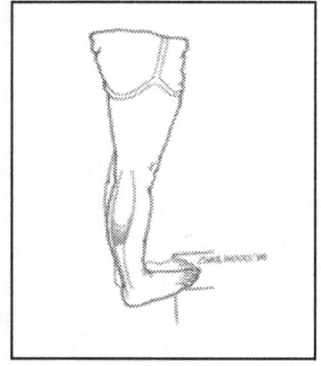

Calf Stretch on Block: Place the balls of your feet on a block or some piece of equipment that will allow you to lean forward while bringing your calves towards the ground. You can sway from side to side while doing this and you'll feel the stretch on the sides of each calf. After swaying a little hold your stretch for ten to thirty seconds.

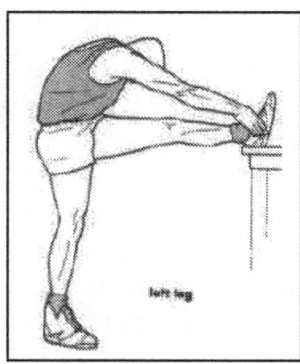

Standing Hamstring Stretch: While standing in front of an object (that you can place your foot on: table, bar, or other piece of equipment) bring one leg up with your knee bent, and rest it on that object. Gradually straighten your knee until it is straight, and go back and forth slowly bending your knee and straightening it. You should feel it stretch the back part of your leg. Perform ten to fifteen of these movements per leg.

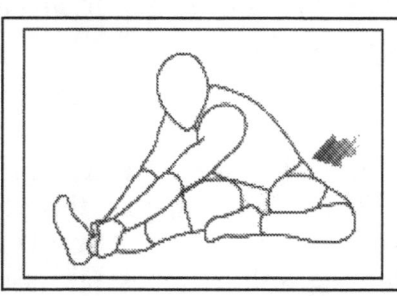

Seated Hamstring Stretch: Sitting on the ground bring one foot into the groin area, and leave the other leg out in front of you. Then slowly lean towards your foot grabbing your ankle to assist in the stretch. Hold this stretch for ten to fifteen seconds and then do the same thing with the other leg.

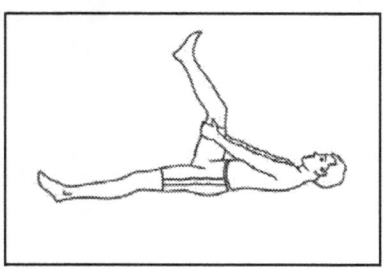

Lying Hamstring Stretch: While lying on the ground bring one leg up while keeping your knee slightly bent. Then grab it with your hands, pulling that leg towards your head. Hold this position for ten to fifteen seconds and then switch to the other leg.

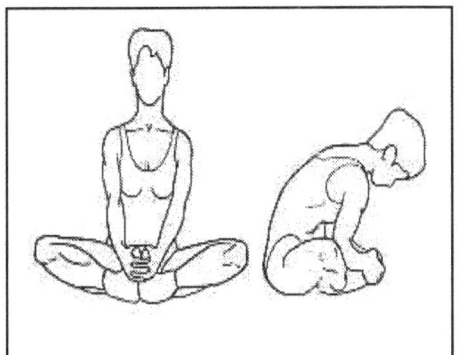

Stationery Groin Stretch: While seated, pull both feet inward toward the body. Grab your feet with your hands, while using the elbows to press downward slightly on the knees. You should feel this stretch in your inner thighs. Hold for 10-30 seconds.

Butterfly Groin Stretch: While in position described above, rock your knees up and down gently stretching your groin area. Rock legs for about ten to fifteen seconds.

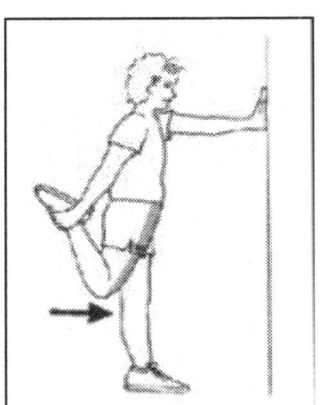

Standing Quadriceps Stretch: While in the standing position grab one foot and pull toward your buttocks, gently stretching your quadriceps. Hold this position for ten to fifteen seconds, and then switch to the other leg. If knee pain occurs discontinue this stretch until problem has been taken care of.

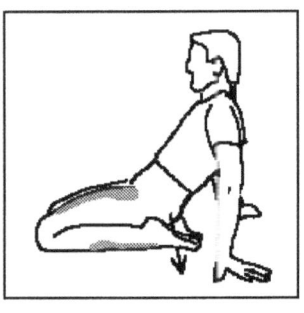

Kneeling Quadriceps Stretch: While sitting on the heels of your feet, or with your heels slightly outside your hip area, lean back until you achieve a full stretch in your quadriceps. Hold this position for ten to thirty seconds. If this position causes discomfort in either knee, discontinue doing it immediately.

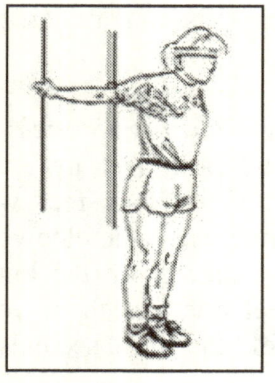

Standing Shoulder Stretch: Grab a bar or piece of equipment and turn away from it gently stretching your shoulder area. Hold stretch for ten to fifteen seconds. You will probably want to perform this with one arm at a time due to the difficulty of doing both arms at one time.

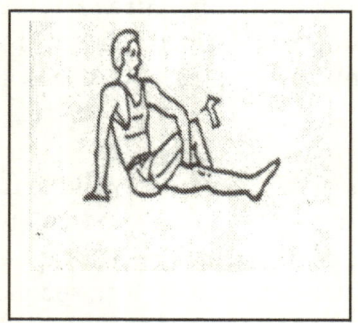

Seated Hip Stretch: While seated on the floor cross one leg over the other leg. Use the opposite arm to press against your knee to feel a stretch in your hip and upper leg. Hold stretch for thirty seconds on each side seconds.

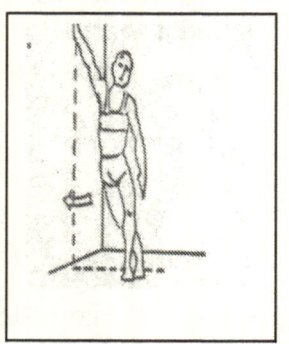

Standing Hip Stretch: Stand sideways at arm's length from a wall. Lean towards the wall with your hip and keep feet firmly on ground. Hold for thirty seconds on each side.

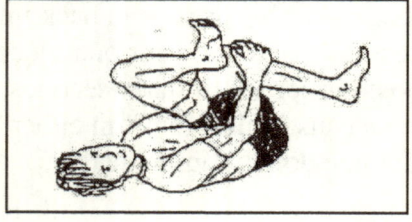

Bent Knee Hip Stretch: While seated place foot/ankle on opposite knee and pull toward chest. This is also an excellent hamstring stretch. Optimal hold time: fifteen to thirty seconds on each side.

165

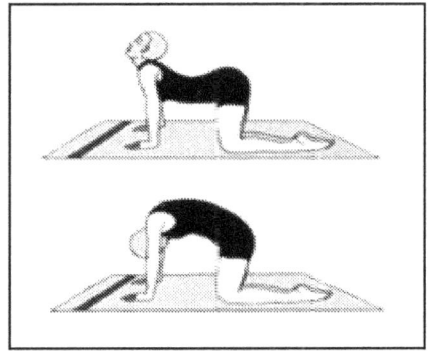

"Cat" (Upper Back) Stretch: To stretch the upper back, hands and knees should be on the floor. Just as a cat would do, slowly lift your back up toward the ceiling dropping your head and shoulders, and rounding your upper back. Hold in place for ten to thirty seconds, or go back and forth in each position for a couple of seconds each. Perform these stretches ten repetitions.

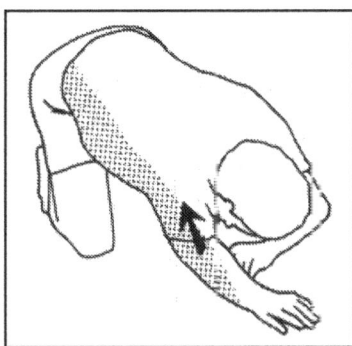

Lower Back Stretch (Baby Position): While kneeling on the floor gently lower your upper body towards the floor. You can leave both arms in front of you for ten seconds; then you can bring both arms back by your sides for ten to thirty seconds. You will be breathing from your diaphragm, due to the position, and with each breath you will feel the stretch in your lower back.

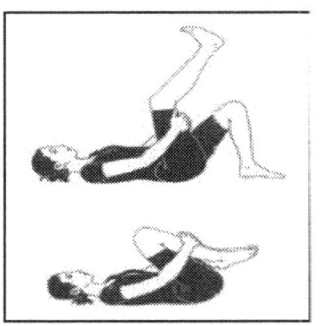

Lower Back Stretch: While lying on your back lift your legs, and with knees bent bring towards your chest; then wrap your arms around your lower legs and gently pull towards your torso. You can do each leg individually and then both legs at the same time. Hold each position for ten to thirty seconds. This is an excellent stretching motion to perform when your back or hamstrings are tight.

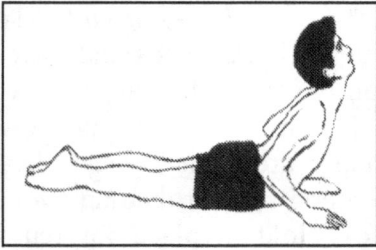

Cobra Stretch: The cobra is a yoga position that is a great lower back stretch. While lying face downward, on the floor, gently raise your upper body to a point where it is arching your back. Hold this position for ten to thirty seconds.

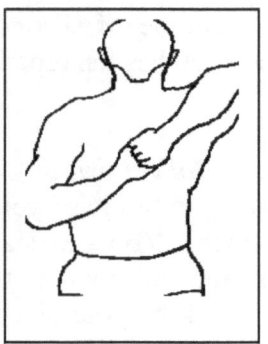

Triceps Stretch: Bend the right arm while placing your fingers in the middle of the back. Using the left arm pull your right elbow backward until you feel the stretch in the back of your arm. If you cannot reach one hand to the other use a canvas strap and hold with the upper hand and grab the strap with the lower hand and continue to stretch the triceps. Hold it for 10-30 seconds. Stretch the other side.

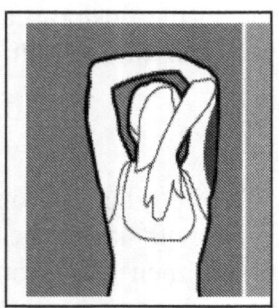

Triceps Stretch: If you cannot perform the stretch listed above try this one. Place one hand behind your middle back area and place the other hand on that elbow. Gently push the arm downward stretching the triceps area of that arm. Then switch arms. Hold position for ten to twenty seconds on each arm.

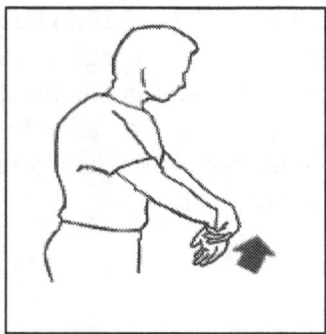

Forearm Stretch: Extend your right arm. Using your left hand, pull your finger tips back toward your body until you feel the stretch in your forearm. Hold the stretch for 10-30 seconds. Repeat using the other arm.

Yoga

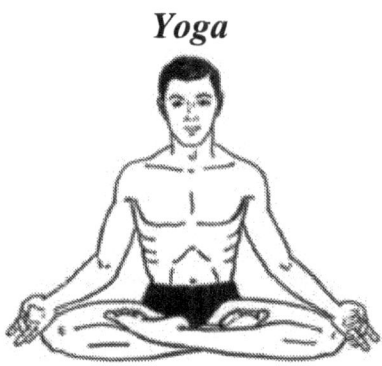

The word "yoga" comes from the Sanskrit word "yuj" which means to unify or to yoke. It involves unifying the mind, body and spirit It originated in northern India more than five thousand years ago Although it is an ancient form of exercise I believe the yoga that is practiced today is one that has evolved to a higher form.

Yoga is an easily adaptive form of exercise that allows the practitioner the option of modifying the movements to meet one's needs. Because of this it is an excellent addition for anyone who is over fifty to add to his or her fitness regime. It can help to increase your flexibility, improve circulation, improve concentration, rejuvenate the mind, and it is valuable in preventing and relieving ailments, such as chronic back pain, arthritis, and migraines.[29]

I've run across people who are afraid to try yoga because they think it is a religious activity. There are many types of yoga, and the one I will be referring to is Hatha Yoga. This form of yoga is simply an advanced system of exercise that can greatly enhance your life. There are a number of different types of Hatha Yoga, and there is one in particular that has gained popularity recently that you probably want to avoid. It is a yoga performed in a very warm room. I have heard people say the temperature may be as hot as one hundred degrees. This can be dangerous to anyone with a hidden condition of high blood pressure.

---

[29] Maran, (2003) Illustrated Yoga, , Thomson Course Technology.

One of the benefits of yoga is that you can do it almost anywhere with a minimal amount of equipment. The basic piece of equipment is the yoga mat. This can be purchased at a discount store for as little as ten dollars. Other pieces of equipment are blocks made of hard rubber, plastic, or wood; canvas straps, and rolled up blankets. These are all relatively inexpensive. To get started all you really require is the mat and some knowledge.

To gain that knowledge you will require some type of instruction. I have learned most of what I know about yoga from books and videos. If you prefer, and you can afford it, an instructor would be the best way to learn. You can get group instruction in a class setting or you can get one on one instruction.

The book that I recommend is *Illustrated Yoga* by Maran. This book has helped me enormously, and I still refer to it often. I recommend starting out by doing the beginner sun salutation. I stayed with this warm-up for approximately two months. During this time I added various movements in the book that I felt I could accomplish and that would benefit me the most. My yoga workout at this point lasted anywhere from ten to twenty minutes.

After getting somewhat proficient at these movements, I began doing the regular sun salutation, and kept adding new movements every now and then. After a couple more months I combined the beginner sun salutation and the regular one to create the one I do now. Once again I want the reader to understand that you should be creative in making a yoga routine that meets all of your needs.

You should never feel like you will not be able to complete your yoga routine because you should have built it like a house. Building your foundation first and then making the room additions is desired. When starting out your movements should be relatively easy. If a movement is difficult, modify it so that you can do it without strain. One of the benefits of yoga is that you can make the positions easy enough for you to be proficient at them, and then as time goes by you can do them with proper positioning in mind.

169

Do not worry if you cannot put your feet behind your head, bend over backwards, or stand on your head for any amount of time. I've been doing yoga for more than one year now and have been involved in fitness for more than thirty years, and there are still many movements that I cannot come close to doing.

Be sure to include a variety of movements. Do some in the standing position, some in the kneeling position, some in an inverted position, (i.e. shoulder stand), and some in the lying position. If you have time try to end your sessions with time in meditation. Meditation scares some people because this is where they think you have to practice some type of Hindu ritual. In reality you can meditate by thinking about your breathing, or in a prayerful state thinking about Jesus. You can even spend time listening to the sounds of silence.

Tai Chi

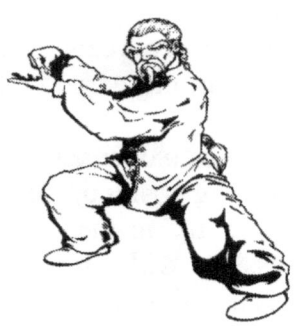

I've included Tai chi under the section on flexibility, although it also increases one's strength and endurance. I have never practiced Tai chi per se, but I do have experience in the martial arts and I can attest to the fact that this is a viable alternative as an adjunct to your fitness regime.

Tai chi (ti-CHE) is sometimes described as "meditation in motion." Originally developed in China as a form of self-defense, this graceful form of exercise has existed for about 2,000 years. It has becoming increasingly popular around the world, both as a basic exercise program and as a complement to other health care methods. In all likelihood this exercise form is used by more people than any other type of exercise form. You could visit parks in China and other countries and find large numbers of participants practicing Tai chi in groups throughout the day.

Tai chi is a noncompetitive, self-paced system of gentle physical exercise. To do Tai chi, you perform a defined series of postures or movements in a slow, graceful manner. Each movement or posture flows into the next without pausing. It is a form of Chinese martial arts which combines deep breathing and relaxation with a number of fundamental postures.

Health benefits include stress reduction, greater balance and increased flexibility; especially important for middle aged (fifty to one hundred year olds) adults. Tai chi hasn't been studied

171

scientifically until recently. Preliminary research shows that for older adults in particular, practicing Tai chi regularly can:

- Reduce anxiety and depression
- Improve balance and coordination, reducing the number of falls
- Improve sleep quality, such as staying asleep longer at night and feeling more alert during the day
- Slow bone loss in women following menopause
- Reduce high blood pressure
- Improve cardiovascular fitness
- Relieve chronic pain
- Improve everyday physical functioning.

Researchers Chen, Collet and Lau recently attempted to determine the effectiveness of Tai chi exercise for people with chronic conditions. They completed a systematic review of forty-seven studies on Tai chi and assessed each study for the effects noted on seven conditions: balance control and falls, musculoskeletal conditions, cardiac and respiratory conditions, psychological responses, endocrine and immune system conditions, and other areas not fitting any of the previous criteria. The results of this analysis appear to link Tai chi to better cardiovascular and respiratory function in patients who have undergone coronary artery bypass surgery, experienced heart failure, or have a history of hypertension or heart attacks. Similar benefits were found for healthy patients who could make Tai chi a beneficial method of prevention for those who are at a high risk for developing heart disease. [30]

Like yoga, there are many styles of Tai chi; some of these styles include: Chen, Hao, Sun, Wu, Yang, Zhao, and Bao.

---

[30] Chenchen Wang, MD; Jean Paul Collet, MD, PhD; Joseph Lau, MD , The Effect of Tai Chi on Health Outcomes in Patients With Chronic Conditions, Archives of Internal.

The intensity of Tai chi varies somewhat depending on the style. For example, the Chen style may be more fast-paced than other styles. However, most styles are gentle and suitable for everyone. Talk to your health care practitioner and Tai chi instructor to make sure the style you're using is appropriate for your physical capabilities.

Balance Training

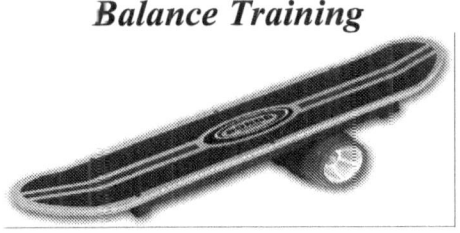

Balance is extremely important in our day to day lives and as we age it becomes even more important. So what exactly is balance, and how can you, the reader work on improving it?

The inner ear balance system works with the eyes, muscles and joints to maintain orientation or balance. For example, visual signals are sent to the brain about the body's position in relation to its surroundings. These signals are processed by the brain, and compared to information from the vestibular and the skeletal systems. Within the inner ear, a complex series of tubes, fluids, and sensitive hairs works to help the brain detect our body's movement and position, including perceptions of up and down, side to side, and circular movements.

While having good balance and sense of body position is a benefit to sports performance, it is critical to preventing falls. Falls among the elderly are a leading cause of debilitating injury (such as hip fractures) and a serious risk factor for premature death. By preventing balance problems and working to improve remaining ability, seniors can improve their quality of life and reduce crippling injuries.

Each year, U.S. hospitals have 300,000 admissions for broken hips, and falling is often the cause of those fractures. Balance exercises can help you stay independent by helping you avoid the disability - often permanent - that may result from falling. Many of you are thinking that this is a bit premature for me to be worrying about at this stage in my life, but if you develop your balance now, it will serve you for the rest of your life.

As you will see, there is a lot of overlap between strength and balance exercises; very often, one exercise serves both purposes.

Any of the lower-body exercises for strength shown in the strength building exercise section also double as balance exercises. Just do your regularly scheduled strength training exercises, yoga movements, tai chi, cardiovascular training exercises, and other flexibility movements and you will improve your balance at the same time. Yoga positions done on one leg are great for enhancing one's ability to balance while strengthening the muscles that assist in balancing.

Good balance is dependent on many different factors, some of them biological, and some of them are capable of improvement. Balance is associated with sensory input from the eyes, the correct functioning of the balance system of the inner ear, and the sense of position and movement in the feet, legs, and arms.

Poor balance can be the side effect of certain medications, medical complications, or serious disorders. For example, dizziness, which can cause difficulty in balancing, can be a result of disease in the vestibular (inner ear balance) system. It can also be due to the side effects of drugs or interactions between different drugs, problems with inadequate or poorly balanced diet, trouble with blood pressure (high or low), or even hyperventilation associated with anxiety.

You can purchase specific equipment to help you develop your balance to a higher degree. These would include balance boards where you stand on a board that has a cylindrical object on the bottom center and it takes an effort to go back and forth while maintaining your balance. Exercising on an exercise ball builds your core muscles and enhances your balance. As mentioned previously, performing one legged positions in yoga or Tai chi will greatly enhance your ability to balance. Try to include one or more of these exercises regularly and you will have a better sense of balance for many years to come!

Putting Your Routine Together

Setting a goal is not the main thing.
It is deciding how you will go about achieving it and staying with
that plan.
Tom Landry, Past Dallas Cowboy Coach

Now it is time to put together a routine for you, the reader. This is the fun and exciting part of the journey. You are about to look and feel better than you have in a long time (unless you're already active and just getting some new ideas). So, let's get started.

The best place to begin is to assess the amount of time you have to spend on your fitness endeavors. Are you going to start off with three days per week (this would be a minimum) or more? Make your assessment realistic; that way you are more apt to do what you plan to do. It will create a positive outcome, instead of one of those resolutions that do not last. If you decided on three days per week you should cover all of the facets of fitness (cardiovascular, strength, and flexibility) on each of these days. If you can start off with four days per week you can do cardio training on two days, and strength training on two days. Your flexibility work should be done with each workout. Remember, this is just our starting point. As I stated earlier the ideal would be to do something seven days per week, but we have to start somewhere, and that somewhere needs to be a realistic place. Always remember that any journey starts with that first step.

At this point you should also commit a certain amount of time per workout. Could you allocate thirty, sixty, or ninety minutes per workout? If thirty minutes is all you can give yourself, then we must make the most of that time, meaning you will be moving at a pretty good pace once you get the hang of things. Sixty or ninety minutes per workout gives you enough time to cover all facets of fitness working in a moderate pace.

After determining this you must decide on whether or not you want to join a fitness center. Ask yourself if you are the type of person that is self-motivated or do you require outside motivation. If you are self-motivated you could probably do all right without joining a fitness center, but if you are not you will make much better gains and enjoy the journey to a higher degree if you join one. Refer back to the section on finding a fitness center to help you make that decision and to help you decide which fitness center you want to join.

Now that you know how much time you will allocate to yourself, and where you will be working out, we can look at the options. The cardiovascular and flexibility training can easily be accomplished without having a gym membership, but the strength training will be accomplished better at a fitness center.

It is generally a good idea to get a complete physical exam from your health practitioner before starting your program. Now let's move forward in our journey.

Some general workout rules to follow are:

- Stop a workout immediately if you feel chest pains or difficulty breathing.
- If you think you have injured yourself stop your workout to check it out.
- Be sure to include something in your weekly program for each facet of fitness: Cardiovascular, strength, and flexibility.
- Always warm up before doing any strenuous activity.
- Always start off by making your workout relatively easy and gentle.
- Make gradual increases with your weights and repetitions.
- Try to make your workouts fun.
- Get a training partner if that is feasible.
- Wear comfortable, loose fitting clothing.
- Never workout right after eating.

- Always keep yourself hydrated by drinking plenty of pure water.
- Be careful when working out outdoors when it is over ninety degrees (including the heat index).
- Never try to impress anyone with your strength and abilities.
- Always ask for help if you are unsure about the correct way to use equipment.
- Keep a workout journal to gauge your progress.
- The recommendations given in this book are to help you create a routine that suits your needs and abilities. It is not set in stone, so improvise when needed.

Three Day Workout

When doing a three day per week workout we will work on all aspects of fitness each of these days. We'll start our routine with our cardiovascular work. I should mention that if you are one of those fortunate people who is trying to gain weight you should do your cardiovascular exercise after your strength training. If you are new at this you can begin with as little as five minutes of cardio as a warm-up. The goal would be to work up to doing twenty to thirty minutes of cardio per workout. You can do a variety of exercises to meet your needs. If you enjoy walking outdoors, then by all means walk outdoors, or if riding on a stationery bike suits you then do that. You have the flexibility to create a routine that you will enjoy and want to do. Pick something from the section on cardio training and do either one each day or switch to a different exercise each day.

If you prefer, you can get your cardio and strength training done together by doing a thing called "Circuit Training." When you circuit train you almost have to work out at a fitness center where they have a group of exercise machines set up for this purpose. You simply go from one machine to another without resting in between until you complete an entire circuit. This may consist of as few as six machines and as many as fifteen machines. After you complete one circuit you may rest for a few minutes and then do one or more circuits, as your physical condition will dictate. This is an excellent way to get in shape, and may be used as a part of a cycle of routines, or on an ongoing basis.

Strength training should be done by working the larger muscle groups first (i.e. legs, back, chest, shoulders, triceps, biceps, and abs) and then work down to the smaller muscle groups. You can start out by doing as few as one set per exercise and work up to three sets per exercise as your body adapts to the workload. Choose one exercise per muscle group from the list given previously. With the larger muscle groups choose an exercise from the list of compound movements for that particular body part, and choose an exercise from the isolation movements when there are no compound movements listed.

Next you will perform your flexibility training as a cool-down from your workout. You should stretch all of the muscle groups as outlined in the section on flexibility, and feel free to choose a particular style of exercise for achieving your flexibility.

When doing a three day per week workout you will alternate days, and perhaps take the weekend off. An example of this would be working out on Monday, Wednesday, and Friday, or doing your workouts on Tuesday, Thursday, and Saturday.

Three Day Workout

- Warm-up with your cardio training.
- Quadriceps exercise: compound movement (leg press machine, or refer to list).
- Upper Back exercise: compound movement (latt pulldowns, or machine rowing).
- Lower Back exercise (hyperextensions, or lower back machine).
- Chest exercise: compound movement (i.e. machine bench press or refer to list of exercises).
- Shoulder exercise: compound movement (i.e. seated machine press or refer to list).

- Triceps exercise: isolation movement: (i.e. triceps extension or refer to list).
- Biceps exercise: isolation movements (any form of curls).
- Abdominal exercise (i.e. crunches, or abdominal machine).
- Flexibility training.

Four Day Workout

Once again we will start with our cardiovascular workout, unless you are trying to gain weight and then you will include it after your strength training. It is a good idea to vary your cardio work when doing a four day workout. You may want to walk one day and use an elliptical training machine the next, or whatever you can conjure up to make your workout experience fun and exciting. As in the previous routine you always want to start off slow and easy and gradually increase the intensity of the workout.

Monday/Thursday & Tuesday/Friday

Monday and Thursday, and Tuesday and Fridays are just the days used as examples. You can change these to fit your schedule. This type of workout is called a split routine because you will be splitting the workout of the various muscles of your body. I like to divide the body into pushing muscles and pulling muscles. Your can divide it other ways such as working the upper or lower body, or working opposing muscle groups (biceps/triceps, chest/back) on the same day.

Here are some sample splits that you can try:

Monday & Thursday
- Warm-up with your cardio training.
- Abdominal exercise: (i.e. crunches, or abdominal machine).
- Lower Back exercise: (hyperextensions, or lower back machine)
- Chest exercise: compound movement (i.e. dumbbell bench press or refer to list of exercises).

180

- Chest exercise: isolation movement (i.e. dumbbell flyes or refer to list).
- Shoulder exercise: compound movement (i.e. seated machine press or refer to list).
- Shoulder exercise: isolation movement (i.e. side lateral raise or refer to list).
- Trap exercise: isolation movement (i.e. shoulder shrug or refer to list).
- Triceps exercise: compound movement (i.e. dips or refers to list).
- Triceps exercise: isolation movement: (i.e. triceps extension or refer to list).
- Flexibility training.

Tuesday and Friday

- Warm-up with your cardio training.
- Abdominal exercise: (i.e. crunches, or abdominal machine).
- Lower Back exercise: (hyperextensions, or lower back machine).
- Upper Back exercise: choose two compound movements (latt pulldowns, and machine rowing or refer to list).
- Biceps exercise: isolation movements (any form of curls).
- Quadriceps exercise: compound movement (leg press machine, or refer to list).
- Quadriceps exercise: isolation movement (leg extensions or refer to list).
- Hamstring exercise: isolation movement (leg curls).
- Calf exercise: isolation movement (any type of calf machine).
- Flexibility training.

Another Four Day Split Workout
(Working Each Muscle Group Once Per Week)

With this type of routine you will be working each muscle group once per week. Because we are giving the muscle lots of time to recuperate we can work it a lot harder than in the other routines. As in the other routines you should start off slow and easy and gradually increase the workload by adding weight, working faster with less rest between sets, or increasing the number of repetitions done.

Monday

- Warm-up with cardio training.
- Abdominal exercise: (i.e. crunches, or abdominal machine).
- Lower Back exercise: (hyperextensions, or lower back machine).
- Chest exercise: two compound movements (refer to list of exercises).
- Chest exercise: isolation movement (refer to list).
- Triceps exercise: compound movement (refer to list of exercises).
- Triceps exercise: isolation movement (refer to list of exercises).
- Flexibility training.

Tuesday

- Warm-up with cardio training.
- Abdominal exercise: (i.e. crunches, or abdominal machine).
- Lower Back exercise: (hyperextensions, or lower back machine).
- Quadriceps exercise: two compound movements (refer to list of exercises).
- Quadriceps exercise: isolation movement (refer to list of exercises).
- Hamstring exercise: isolation movement (leg curls).
- Calf exercise: two isolation movements (any two calf exercises on the list).
- Flexibility training.

Thursday

- Warm-up with cardio training.
- Abdominal exercise: (i.e. crunches, or abdominal machine).
- Lower Back exercise: (hyperextensions, or lower back machine).
- Upper Back exercise: choose three compound movements (latt pulldowns, and machine rowing and refer to list of exercises).
- Biceps exercise: two isolation movements (any form of curls from list).
- Flexibility training.

Friday

- Warm-up with cardio training.
- Abdominal exercise: (i.e. crunches, or abdominal machine).
- Lower Back exercise: (hyperextensions, or lower back machine).
- Shoulder exercise: two compound movements (refer to list of exercises).
- Shoulder exercise: two isolation movements (refer to list of exercises).
- Trap exercise: isolation movement (i.e. shoulder shrug or refer to list).
- Flexibility training.

Remember these routines are samples of what you could incorporate, but they are not the only routines you could follow to get great results. Utilize the time and equipment you have at your disposal to your best advantage. Always keep in mind that the key to continuous progress is to gradually increase resistance applied to the muscles, reducing rest time between sets, and increasing repetitions when applicable. I apologize for being redundant at times, but it is important to follow some of these basic concepts that are being drilled into you.

Training Setbacks

Humans are habitual. They strive on routine and rituals. While it's true that routine can provide a sense of ease and security, I think we'd all agree that the same old, same old could also turn to boredom. And when it comes to working out, routine can be downright toxic.

New exercisers often see quick fitness results such as weight loss and increased muscle strength while engaging in the same workout day after day. However, after several weeks following their fitness routines they often become frustrated as the gains begin to dwindle. Eventually dieters' scales become frozen on the same number, or weight lifters are stuck at the same weights. They hit a plateau.

A plateau typically is the direct consequence of a fitness rut – when an exerciser performs the same workout over and over. The human body is very efficient and quickly adapts to work. Once the body practices the same activity repeatedly, it grows more proficient at performing those moves. So that means it requires less energy and therefore also burns fewer calories.

Instead of celebrating their body's improved fitness capabilities, exercisers often abandon their workouts. And who can blame them? After all, they no longer are seeing the results they desire and become increasingly bored with their workouts. Plus, hitting a plateau not only can halt fitness gains, but it can even reverse previous successes. With just a few simple steps, exercisers can easily break-through that brick wall and continue to reap all the rewards of regular physical activity.

Dodging the dreaded plateau is actually very easy. Variety is the key ingredient to continual fitness success. To avoid hitting a workout plateau, follow these recommendations.

To begin with, every workout routine should be changed about every four to six weeks. The modification doesn't have to be dramatic. A totally new exercise is a possible option, but alteration of a current exercise can be just as effective.

A simple way to determine how to transform your current workout is using the F.I.T.T principle. F.I.T.T. stands for frequency, intensity, time and type. This strategy can be adopted for both cardio and resistance-training.

Frequency: Increase or decrease how often you workout.

Intensity: Increase or decrease the difficulty or level at which you workout.

Time: Increase or decrease how long your workout sessions last.

Type: Change the type of exercises you perform.

Frequency and Time are limited by an individual's schedule as well as appropriate rest time to ensure maximum efficiency and safety. Intensity and Type are really only limited by creativity and planning.

Cardio exercise intensity can easily be varied through speed, incline, distance, etc.; and of course the types of exercises are practically endless, so exercisers should never have the excuse that they've exhausted their exercise options. Good cardio examples include: walking, jogging, swimming, biking, hiking, rebounding, and more. In addition, combining several of these exercises into one workout session can be very effective. Try ten minutes each of three to four unique exercises.

Strength training intensity can also easily be altered with changes in resistance amounts, number of reps, rest time, number of sets and more. Even simply switching the sequence of the exercises can prove effective. There are also numerous strength training exercise options. Unfortunately, most exercisers are unaware of the variety of training techniques and equipment options.

They often get stuck performing the same eight to ten exercises over and over. Yet, there are hundreds of unique options. Simply utilizing new types of training equipment every four to six weeks can result in big improvements because each type of equipment will work the muscle groups in a slightly different manner. Equipment options include: free weights, machines, body bars, resistance bands and tubing, and fitness balls – just to name a few.

So, to reduce your chances of hitting a plateau remember the F.I.T.T. principle; and approximately every four to six weeks choose one element of the principle to change (or even all four components). Incorporating this strategy will enable you to progress further and attain even higher fitness levels. It's just that easy, or is it?

Even when you usually enjoy exercising, there will be days when you just can't seem to find the motivation to get active. Here are some practical tips to help keep up enthusiasm.

Keep a diary. Whatever sport or activity you do, this can help you. Write down how far you ran or the match score, your pulse, how you felt etc. That way you can look back and see how you have improved over time.

Collect inspiration. Stick quotes from coaches, athletes, or anyone successful around your house and/or your office. Inspirational stories from people who have achieved against the odds may help - if they can do it, so can you!

When it comes to staying motivated it's just as important to train your brain as it is to train your body. Here are just a few ideas to help you win the mental battle and stay on the exercise track.

Set yourself some short and long-term goals. Success will provide you with a sense of satisfaction and further motivation to keep up the new lifestyle. Keep your goals SMART:

Specific Goals
Measurable Goals
Achievable Goals
Realistic Goals
Time-based Goals.

For example, rather than saying you'll get fit by summer, start by setting the more specific goal of going to an hour-long fitness class every week, or doing just five minutes of exercise every day.

A great way to stay focused is to keep reminding yourself of the reasons that motivated you to start exercising in the first place, such as the aim of losing weight, improving your health, attracting someone special for a date, or testing yourself by competing in a race (either walking, running, biking, or swimming).

Visualization is a powerful technique used by professional athletes to perform at their best. Picture yourself achieving your goal, such as completing a race or slipping into the next size down in a dress or trousers, and imagine what it will feel like. These images and feelings will help to motivate you to achieving them for real.

Enjoy it! Exercising releases chemicals in the brain, such as serotonin, that have a strong affect on your mood, helping reduce anxiety, stress and depression. So whenever you don't feel like exercising, try to remind yourself how good you'll feel afterwards. I can remember many times when I didn't really feel like going to the gym for a workout, but I also remember that I felt so much better each and every time that I did go and workout. Once at the gym I started to feel more energetic already, and don't forget that it is actually difficult to feel depressed after a vigorous workout. That's right--you will almost have to try to be depressed if that's what you want!

It is also pleasant to make friends at the local fitness center or join a club where members enjoy the same activity as you. Knowing that people will ask for you if you are not present or call you when you miss a session is also beneficial. This too can help you stick to your fitness regime.

It's just like going to the local pub like in the sitcom, "Cheers", which illustrated how friendships can be formed outside the family or workplace.

n life there will be setbacks and disappointments. Your journey towards achieving health and fitness will be no different. It reminds me of the story of Nicolo Paganini who was a well-known and gifted nineteenth century violinist. He was also well known as a great showman with a quick sense of humor. His most memorable concert was in Italy with a full orchestra. He was performing before a packed house, and his technique was incredible, his tone was fantastic, and his audience dearly loved him. Toward the end of his concert, Paganini was astounding his audience with an unbelievable composition when suddenly one string on his violin snapped and hung limply from his instrument. Paganini frowned briefly, shook his head, and continued to play, improvising beautifully.

Then to everyone's surprise, a second string broke, and shortly thereafter, a third. Almost like a slapstick comedy, Paganini stood there with three strings dangling from his Stradivarius. But instead of leaving the stage, Paganini stood his ground and calmly completed the difficult number on the one remaining string.

Please do not ever give up. If you persevere you will get past those trying times. When you feel as though three of your four strings have broken, you can continue on. You can and will achieve health and fitness if you just hang in there!

My Personal Fitness Regime

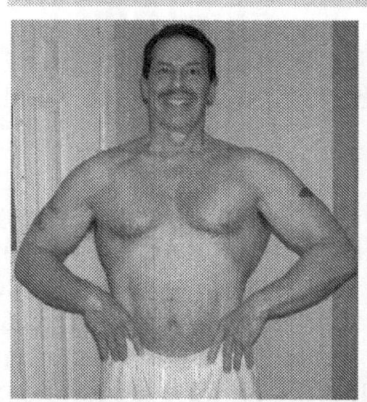

I've been an exercise enthusiast for most of my life. I am probably an exception to the rule because I must admit that I enjoy most of my fitness endeavors. The reason I say "most" instead of "all" is because I too have days when it is a chore to go through the motions of exercise. Fortunately for me, they are few and far between. The reason I can enjoy my fitness endeavors is because I have chosen the ones that I like to do. It is never a good idea to embark on a fitness program doing things you know you hate to do. For that reason I want you, the reader, to pick and choose the activities that you are most apt to stick with for long periods of time.

As we go through life and take a journey in fitness we will change our direction from time to time. This if perfectly all right! The key is to continually do something. Just keep moving, even if you are moving slowly.

Listed below are the fitness endeavors that I am currently doing. This may change next week or next month, but this is my current training regime.

Yoga

At the present time I start each day with thirty minutes of yoga. I started doing yoga about one and a half years ago, and I must admit I really enjoy it. The benefits are tremendous. When I decided to start doing yoga I looked at a variety of books and found one called Illustrated Yoga. It worked well for me because it had lots of pictures as the title implies. After purchasing the book I then purchased a yoga mat. You can get these at discount stores for as little as ten dollars. That's about all it takes to get started.

Of course you could take classes from a professional if this is the best way for you to learn how to do it and to keep you motivated.

I started off by doing a modified "Sun Salutation." The sun salutation is designed to arm the body in preparation for the rest of the workout. When I first started I did the beginner's version of the sun salutation (outlined in detail in the above mentioned book) for as little as five minutes per session. This was my entire yoga workout. I think it is important to ease into fitness endeavors. That way we can avoid injuring ourselves, and it makes the whole endeavor more pleasant. I gradually added movements and added more rounds of the sun salutation as I went along.

I then went to the regular version of the sun salutation. After a while I combined some of both and even added a couple of other moves. Yoga is a highly individualized exercise form. You can modify the moves; their order, and the duration of time each one is held to suit your needs. As I became more proficient at the moves I added more difficult ones. This taxed my abilities, but was never a task that I thought I might not be able to perform.

Today I perform the modified sun salutation fifteen times, and then I do a variety of other moves for a total of a thirty-minute session. When designing a yoga workout you must adhere to the general principles outlined earlier.

My Cardio Training

Walking, in my opinion, is one of the best exercises a person over fifty can do. I get my walking in by walking to and from the fitness center. This kills two or more birds with one stone. First it gives me time outdoors to breathe fresh air and enjoy the scenery. Second it gets me to the gym without using that precious commodity, gasoline.

In the past I would do cardiovascular work after my weight training, but now I incorporate walking as my cardio training. On days when the weather does not permit me to walk I will do twenty minutes of cardio on one of the cardio machines in the gym (treadmill, stair climber, recumbent bike, etc.).

Rebounding

Approximately three evenings per week I do ten to thirty minutes of rebounding on a mini trampoline. It's a relatively easy form of exercise and it places very little stress on the joints. I start out by bouncing (without leaving the rebounder) for about five minutes as a form of warm-up; and then I jog, or walk in place for the rest of the time, with occasional breaks to bounce. I do this while watching television, and the time goes by rapidly.

My Weight Training

I generally cycle my weight training by doing a full body workout for four to six weeks; a split routine for four to six weeks, and a further split routine for four to six weeks. Please refer to the explanation on how to do each exercise that was given previously.

Full Body Routines

When I do my full body workouts I usually start off by doing a couple of weeks of circuit training. Circuit training is when you go from one piece of equipment to another without any rest in between. Most fitness centers are set up with one or more areas for circuit training. You simply go down the line of equipment doing one set of each one. I usually go around the circuit three times. This gives me work in a cardiovascular manner at the same time as strength training.

After two weeks of circuit training I will perform my full body workout by working the largest muscle groups first. I do full body workouts three times per week. This workout looks like this:

Warm-up: Walk to my fitness center, or 20 minutes of cardio on one of the machines.
Core Muscle Work: Crunches: 100 Reps; Hyperextensions: 40 Reps; Leg Raise: 2 X 20.
Leg Press: 3 sets of 8 – 12 reps.
Leg Extensions: 3 X 8-12.
Leg Curls: 3 X 8-12.
Heel Raise: 3 X 10-20.
Machine Rows: 3 X 8-12.
Machine Bench Press: 3 X 8-12.
Seated Press: 3 X 8-12.
Shrugs: 3 X 8-12.
Curls: 3 X 8-12.
Triceps Pushdown: 3 X 8-12.
Stretch: 15 minutes
Walk home

Split Routine

I like to do what is known as a push/pull split routine. What this means is that I do the pushing muscles (chest, shoulders, and triceps) on one day. Then I do the pulling muscles (back, and biceps) and also legs on the next day. I do this on Monday, Tuesday, Thursday and Friday. This works each muscle group two times per week. This workout looks like this:

Monday/Thursday
Chest/Shoulders/Triceps

Warm-up: Walk to the gym, or do cardio on a machine at the gym.
Core Muscle Work: Crunches: 100 Reps; Hyperextensions: 40 Reps; Leg Raise: 2 X 20.
Machine Dips: 4 X 8-12 (warm-up for chest/triceps).
Hammer Strength Bench Press Machine: 4 X 8-12.

Machine Flyes: 4 X 8-12.
Seated Rear Delt Machine: 4 X 8-12.
Machine Shoulder Press: 4 X 8-12.
Shrugs: 4 X 8-12.
Dumbbell Triceps Extension: 4 X 8-12.
Triceps Pushdowns (on Latt Machine): 4 X 8-12.
Stretch: 15 Minutes
Walk home.

Tuesday/Friday
Legs/Back/Biceps

Warm-up: Walk to the gym, or do cardio on a machine at the gym.
Core Muscle Work: Crunches: 100 Reps; Hyperextensions: 40 Reps;
Leg Raise: 2 X 20.
Seated Machine Rows: 4 X 8-12.
Latt Pulldowns: 4 X 8-12.
Hammer Strength Machine Curls: 4 X 8-12.
Leg Press (one leg at a time): 4 X 8-12.
Leg Extension: 4 X 8-12.
Leg Curl: 4 X 8-12.
Seated Heel Raise (Bent Knee): 4 X 8-12.
Calf Machine: 4 X 8-12.
Stretch: 15 Minutes
Walk home.

Further Split Routine

During this phase of my training I split my routine even further and work each muscle group one time per week, doing a higher intensity workout for each muscle group. This is also done four days per week as follows:

Monday
Chest/Triceps

Warm-up: Walk to the gym, or do cardio on a machine at the gym.

Core Muscle Work: Crunches: 100 Reps; Hyperextensions: 40 Reps;
Leg Raise: 2 X 20.
Machine Dips: 4 X 8-12.
Flat Bench Press (Hammer Strength Machine): 4 X 8-12.
Incline Bench Press (Hammer Strength Machine): 4 X 8-12.
Flyes (Machine): 4 X 8-12.
Triceps Extensions (Dumbbell): 4 X 8-12.
Triceps Pushdowns (Cable): 4 X 8-12.
Stretch: 15 Minutes
Walk home.

Tuesday
Back/Biceps/Forearms

Core Muscle Work: Crunches: 100 Reps; Hyperextensions: 40 Reps;
Leg Raise: 2 X 20.
One Arm Rowing (Hammer Strength Machine): 4 X 8-12.
Reverse Grip Pulldowns (Hammer Strength Machine): 4 X 8-12.
Latt Pulldowns (Cable): 4 X 8-12.
Curls (Hammer Strength Machine): 4 X 8-12.
Alternate Dumbbell Curls: 4 X 8-12.
Wrist Curls (Barbell): 4 X 8-12.
Stretch: 15 Minutes
Walk home.

Thursday
Legs

Core Muscle Work: Crunches: 100 Reps; Hyperextensions: 40 Reps;
Leg Raise: 2 X 20.
Machine Squat (Hammer Strength Machine): 4 X 8-12.
Lunges: 4 X 8-12.
Leg Extensions: 4 X 8-12.
Standing Leg Curls (Machine): 4 X 8-12.
Seated Heel Raise: 4 X 8-12.
Heel Raise (Hammer Strength Machine): 4 X 8-12.

Stretch: 15 Minutes
Walk home.

Friday
Shoulders/Traps

Core Muscle Work: Crunches: 100 Reps; Hyperextensions: 40 Reps;
Leg Raise: 2 X 20.
Rear Lateral Raise (Machine): 4 X 8-12.
Seated Shoulder Press Machine: 4 X 8-12.
Side Lateral Raise (Dumbbells): 4 X 8-12.
Upright Rowing (Barbell): 4 X 8-12.
Shrugs: 4 X 8-12.
Stretch: 15 Minutes
Walk home.

There are many ways to accomplish the goal of achieving health and fitness for the over fifty group. I have given you my personal regime, and some general workouts and guidelines, but let's be open minded and remember there is a best way to achieve this, and the best way will be slightly different for each of us.

According to *Prevention Magazine*, getting back to a younger body takes the following:
- Incorporate a healthy low-fat, low-calorie, high fiber, diet.
- Do at least 45 minutes a day of some kind of moderate aerobic activity.
- Emphasis should be placed on resistance training to build muscle mass.

As you can see my personal view is somewhat different from that of *Prevention Magazine*, but their position would help a person achieve health and fitness. It is a matter of finding what works best for your physiology, time constraints, and level of desire.

Knowledge is power, and the more you possess concerning health and fitness, the better off you will be. Read about health and fitness regularly for a number of reasons. First, it gives you the knowledge to make decisions concerning your routines, and secondly it will serve to motivate you on an ongoing basis.

What to Do if Injury Occurs

For the over fifty group certain injuries are more common because of age and physical condition. These include degenerative arthritis, muscle sprains and strains, and lower back pain and tendonitis. Injuries can occur through various circumstances: accidents, inexperience, carelessness, and most commonly, poor form and excess repetitions and sets.

If an injury such as a strain or sprain occurs, people have access to a four-part approach known as RICE: Rest, Ice, Compression and Elevation. Utilizing this process will improve the chance of a faster and more complete recovery.

- Rest: Resting the body, and more importantly, the area of injury, is critical for the body to repair itself. The amount of resting varies from one person to the next; each person's injury and recuperation time are unique.
- Ice: Providing pain relief, ice can significantly reduce swelling on the injured body part. You should leave ice on the injury for no more than twenty or twenty-five minutes. In haste to speed the process, however, you may be tempted to leave the ice on the injury longer. But doing so can damage the skin and tissue.
- Compression: Minimizing swelling, compression aids in healing the injured body part. You should wrap an ACE bandage over the injury, using a figure-8 wrapping technique. If the wrap feels too tight, remove and rewrap for a more comfortable feel.
- Elevation: The last part of the healing process, elevation reduces swelling. You should raise the injured area above the level of the heart and prop the injured body part on pillows to maximize comfort.

Along with RICE, you can gently stretch and massage the injured area for fast recovery. Although RICE is a commonly used procedure with a high success rate, the process is not foolproof. If the pain and swelling remain severe or persist for more than forty-eight hours, you should see a physician.

Minor injuries typically last one to two weeks, but a severe injury can last several weeks. In general, a minor injury, such as a mild sprain, causes overstretching or slight tearing of the ligaments with no joint instability. Someone with a mild sprain usually experiences minimal pain, swelling and a minor loss of functional ability. Sprains of greater severity cause partial tearing of the ligament and are characterized by bruising and swelling. Someone with a severe sprain usually experiences some or total loss of function.

If you feel as though your back may be out from its normal position, you should let a reputable chiropractor realign it by using manual adjustments. By getting regular adjustments you could keep your back in its proper alignment and avoid potential back injuries.

It is also a good idea to see a chiropractor as soon as possible after a back or neck injury. Refer to the section on back injuries for more information.

Middle aged people (fifty to one hundred year olds) have the chance to maintain their lives through physical activity. By implementing the program outlined in this book and adhering to a healthy diet, you will place yourself on the right path for enjoying your middle and latter years of life as much as you have the years preceding them.

Possible Health Problems & Solutions

It doesn't matter how many times you get knocked down in life as long as you get up just one more time than you were knocked down!
Steve Fisher, ND

Even a healthy and fit person will encounter health problems during his or her lifetime. It is a perfectly normal occurrence to injure a muscle or strain a ligament when you are pursuing a lifestyle of health and fitness. When these challenges occur it is important to have the knowledge to deal with them in the most effective manner possible. This book will give you some of that knowledge to incorporate into your life.

Let's continue our journey and gain some of the knowledge needed to handle what life has to throw at us.

Back Injuries

Back pain is an all-too-familiar problem that can range from a dull, constant ache to a sudden, sharp pain that leaves you incapacitated. It can come on suddenly from an accident, a fall, or lifting something too heavy or it can develop slowly, perhaps as the result of age-related changes to the spine. Regardless of how it happens or how it feels, you know it when you have it. And chances are if you don't have it now, you will experience some form of it eventually.

At some point, back pain affects an estimated eight out of ten people. It is one of our society's most common medical problems. Although anyone can have back pain, a number of factors increase your risk. They include:

Age: The first attack of low back pain typically occurs between the ages of thirty and forty. Back pain becomes more common with age.

Fitness level: Back pain is more common among people who are not physically fit. Weak back and abdominal muscles may not properly support the spine. "Weekend warriors" (people who go out and exercise a lot after being inactive all week) are more likely to suffer painful back injuries than people who make moderate physical activity a daily habit. Studies show that low-impact aerobic exercise is good for the discs that cushion the vertebrae, the individual bones that make up the spine.

Diet: A diet high in calories and fat, combined with an inactive lifestyle, can lead to obesity, which can put stress on the back.

Heredity: Some causes of back pain, including disc disease, may have a genetic component.

Race: Race can be a factor in back problems. African American women, for example, are two to three times more likely than white women to develop spondylolisthesis, a condition in which a vertebra of the lower spine, also called the lumbar spine, slips out of place.

The presence of other diseases: Many diseases can cause or contribute to back pain. These include various forms of arthritis, such as osteoarthritis, rheumatoid arthritis, and ankylosing spondylitis, and cancers elsewhere in the body that may spread to the spine.

Occupational risk factors: Having a job that requires heavy lifting, pushing or pulling, particularly when this involves twisting or vibrating the spine, can lead to injury and back pain. An inactive job or a desk job may also lead to or contribute to pain, especially if you have poor posture or sit all day in an uncomfortable chair.

Cigarette smoking: Although smoking may not directly cause back pain, it increases your risk of developing low back pain and low back pain with sciatica. (Sciatica is back pain that radiates to the hip and/or leg due to pressure on a nerve.) For example, smoking may lead to pain by blocking your body's ability to deliver nutrients to the discs of the lower back. Or, repeated coughing due to heavy smoking may cause back pain. It is also possible that smokers are just less physically fit or less healthy than nonsmokers, which increases the likelihood that they will develop back pain. Furthermore, smoking can slow healing, prolonging pain for people who have had back injuries, back surgery, or broken bones.

It is important to understand that back pain is a symptom of a medical condition, not a diagnosis itself. Medical problems that can cause back pain include the following:

Mechanical problems: A mechanical problem is a problem with the way your spine moves or the way you feel when you move your spine in certain ways. Perhaps the most common mechanical cause of back pain is a condition called intervertebral disc degeneration, which simply means that the discs located between the vertebrae of the spine are breaking down with age. As they deteriorate, they lose their cushioning ability. This problem can lead to pain if the back is stressed. Other mechanical causes of back pain include spasms,

201

muscle tension, and ruptured discs, which are also called herniated discs.

Injuries: Spine injuries such as sprains and fractures can cause either short-lived or chronic pain. Sprains are tears in the ligaments that support the spine, and they can occur from twisting or lifting improperly. Fractured vertebrae are often the result of osteoporosis, a condition that causes weak, porous bones. Less commonly, back pain may be caused by more severe injuries that result from accidents and falls.

Acquired conditions and diseases: Many medical problems can cause or contribute to back pain. They include scoliosis, which causes curvature of the spine and does not usually cause pain until mid-life; spondylolisthesis; various forms of arthritis, including osteoarthritis, rheumatoid arthritis, and ankylosing spondylitis; and spinal stenosis, a narrowing of the spinal column that puts pressure on the spinal cord and nerves. While osteoporosis itself is not painful, it can lead to painful fractures of the vertebrae. Other causes of back pain include pregnancy; kidney stones or infections; endometriosis, which is the buildup of uterine tissue in places outside the uterus, and fibromyalgia, which causes fatigue and widespread muscle pain.

Infections and tumors: Although they are not common causes of back pain, infections can cause pain when they involve the vertebrae, a condition called osteomyelitis, or when they involve the discs that cushion the vertebrae, which is called discitis. Tumors, too, are relatively rare causes of back pain. Occasionally, tumors begin in the back, but more often they appear in the back as a result of cancer that has spread from elsewhere in the body.

Although the causes of back pain are usually physical, it is important to know that emotional stress can play a role in how severe pain is and how long it lasts. Stress can affect the body in many ways, including causing back muscles to become tense and painful.

Eating a healthy diet also is important. For one thing, eating to maintain a healthy weight or to lose weight, if you are overweight, helps you avoid putting unnecessary and injury-causing stress and strain on your back. To keep your spine strong, as with all bones, you need to get enough calcium, magnesium and vitamin D every day. These nutrients help prevent osteoporosis, which is responsible for a lot of the bone fractures that lead to back pain. Calcium is found in dairy products, green, leafy vegetables, and fortified products, like orange juice. Your skin makes vitamin D when you are in the sun. If you are not outside much, you can obtain vitamin D from your diet, almost all milk and some other foods are fortified with this nutrient. Most adults don't get enough calcium and vitamin D, so talk to your doctor about how much you need per day, and consider taking a nutritional supplement or a multivitamin.

Practicing good posture, supporting your back properly, and avoiding heavy lifting when you can may all help you prevent injury. If you do lift something heavy, keep your back straight. Don't bend over the item; instead, lift it by putting the stress on your legs and hips.

I can speak from personal experience when I say that a back injury can cause excruciating pain and recurrent problems. The first time I injured my back was in the 1970s when I was powerlifting. Powerlifting is the sport of lifting as heavy a weight as possible in three different lifts (squat, bench press and dead lift). All three of these motions are possible injuries waiting to happen. Yes, this sounds like a dumb thing to do, but when you're in your twenties you feel invincible and do some pretty dumb things. My problem began after squatting (placing an Olympic style barbell on the upper back behind your neck and bending your knees until your hamstrings are breaking the point of being parallel to the ground) a heavy weight during a training session.

While lowering my upper body I hit a place where my hip felt as though it was out of place. It sounded as though someone had shot me, and my legs went out from under me. I was diagnosed with a pelvic tilt, and one leg was now slightly longer than the other. I was the owner and operator of a fitness center at this time, thus I was able to take some time off to recover. It seems as though for a long time my back would give me problems every now and then. I can remember times when I had to grab a wall to get to the bathroom, or crawl on the floor to get into the right position to get up.

I found that chiropractic adjustments gave me a lot of relief and would place my spine and hip joints back into a correct position. Unfortunately they wouldn't always stay there. I also tried acupuncture and this too gave me some relief.

As I got a little older and hopefully wiser I avoided the high-risk exercises such as the squat and deadlift, and the problem occurred less frequently. Something that I had neglected over the years was the area of flexibility. After turning fifty I began to concentrate more on this area of fitness, and I learned that I was not very flexible. Approximately one and a half years ago I incorporated yoga into my daily routine, and this has helped me immensely. If I do get a spasm in my back, it is never as severe and doesn't last as long. I recommend that everyone over fifty do yoga on a regular basis. You will find more about yoga in the section on exercise.

I've also learned to use nutritional products to aid me. I use bromelain, which comes from pineapple, on a daily basis. Bromelain is one of the best natural anti-inflammatory nutrients around. I also use ginger, and boswellia, which also act as a natural anti-inflammatory; Glucosamine, Chondroitan, and MSM, which are sulfates that lubricate, add fluid to joints, and decrease pain in joints. I also take extra Vitamin C in the form of Ester-C (500mg capsules 2-3 times per day).

Something that I have never heard of helping a back injury was introduced to me by one of my clients (which goes to show you that we can always learn something from other people) is creatine. I had taken creatine on and off to improve the muscles' appearance, but never realized it was helping my back, so I experimented with myself and found it worked really well for me. Now I recommend a teaspoon of pure creatine monohydrate per day to all my clients with back injuries.

Walking is an excellent form of exercise, especially for those with a back problem. Start out slow and easy and gradually add distance and speed to your walking regime. You can find more about walking in the section on exercise.

Treating Back Injuries in a Nutshell

- During the first twenty-four to forty-eight hours apply ice to a muscle spasm.
- Always drink lots of pure water (at least 64 oz. per day).
- Rest the injured area for twenty-four hours.
- Bromelain: 500 Mg. 2 – 3 times per day.
- Creatine Monohydrate (pure form with no flavoring): 1 teaspoon per day.
- Glucosamine Sulfate: 1500 mg. per day
- Chondroitan Sulfate: 500 mg. per day
- MSM as needed for pain.
- Be certain you are getting adequate nutrition on a daily basis. With emphasis on plenty of calcium (1500 mg per day), magnesium (800 mg. per day), Vitamin D (400 IU per day), B-12 (200 mcg. per day), and a good whole food multi-vitamin/mineral supplement.
- Light stretching as soon as possible. Be sure to do this without pain. If pain persists stop immediately.
- Walking as soon as possible to prevent pain.
- Begin a yoga program designed to help back problems and do on a daily basis.

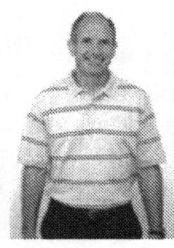

Joseph Y. is a chiropractor and acupuncturist who practices what he preaches. He is an extremely healthy looking individual who seems to do all the right things regarding health and fitness. He attributes his good health to his lifestyle of eating correctly, exercising regularly, resting and having a positive mental attitude. He attributes his high degree of fitness to high intensity, low volume, short duration exercise using resistance and interval training, which is followed by flexibility work and rest.

His exercise regime includes two days a week doing interval training in which he sprints, and two days a week of free weight strength training with concentration on the core muscles using balance boards and plyometrics.

He balances his protein and carbohydrate intake, while avoiding refined carbohydrates such as white sugar. Joseph eats vegetables freely, includes two fruits a day in his diet, eats nuts and olive oil, and drinks mineral spring water. He supplements his diet with multi-vitamins/minerals/trace minerals, magnesium, sulfur, mixed vitamin E, alpha lipoic acid, and Carnitine betaine, And Co Q-10.

Stress is dealt with exercise, breathing techniques, and a positive mental attitude. He doesn't use any pharmaceutical drugs on a regular basis, nor does he smoke or use any tobacco products. On occasions, which are every three to four months, he will drink some wine or beer.

Joseph, like me, believes that people should live to one hundred and ten to one hundred and twenty years. He doesn't expect to see a decline in his health or fitness levels until he reaches ninety.

Knee Problems

Mechanical knee problems can be caused by: A direct blow or sudden movements that strain the knee, and osteoarthritis in the knee, resulting from wear and tear on its parts. Inflammatory knee problems can be caused by certain rheumatic diseases, such as rheumatoid arthritis and systemic lupus erythematosus (lupus). These diseases cause swelling which can damage the knees permanently.

The most common type of arthritis of the knee is osteoarthritis. In this disease, the cartilage in the knee gradually wears away. Treatments for osteoarthritis are: acupuncture, physical therapy, anti-inflammatory products, fish oil, glucosamine, chondroitan, microlactin, creatine, and exercises to improve movement and strength and weight loss.

Rheumatoid arthritis is another type of arthritis that affects the knee. In rheumatoid arthritis, the knee becomes inflamed and cartilage may be destroyed. Treatment for this disease includes: Physical therapy, fish oil, natural anti-inflammatory herbs and enzymes, dietary changes, possible medications, and possibly knee replacement surgery (for a seriously damaged knee).

Cartilage Injuries and Disorders

Chondromalacia (KON-dro-muh-lay-she-uh) occurs when the cartilage of the knee cap softens. This can be caused by injury, overuse, or muscle weakness, or if parts of the knee are out of alignment. Chondromalacia can develop if a blow to the knee cap tears off a piece of cartilage or a piece of cartilage containing a bone fragment.

The meniscus (meh-NISS-kus) is a C-shaped piece of cartilage that acts like a pad between the femur (thigh bone) and tibia (shin bone). It is easily injured if the knee is twisted while bearing weight. A partial or total tear may occur. If the tear is tiny, the meniscus stays connected to the front and back of the knee. If the tear is large, the meniscus may be left hanging by a thread of cartilage. The seriousness of the injury depends on the location and the size of the tear.

Treatment for cartilage injuries includes: Exercises to strengthen muscles, electrical stimulation to strengthen muscles, dietary changes, natural anti-inflammatory herbs and enzymes, and surgery for severe injuries.

Ligament Injuries

Two commonly injured ligaments in the knee are the anterior cruciate ligament (ACL) and the posterior cruciate ligament (PCL). An injury to these ligaments is sometimes called a "sprain." The ACL is most often stretched or torn (or both) by a sudden twisting motion. The PCL is usually injured by a direct impact, such as in an automobile accident or football tackle.

A blow to the outer side of the knee usually injures the medial and lateral collateral ligaments. This can stretch and tear a ligament. These blows frequently occur in sports such as football or hockey.

Ligament injuries are treated with: Ice packs (right after the injury) to reduce swelling, exercises to strengthen muscles, use of a brace, natural anti inflammatory herbs and enzymes, and possibly surgery (for more severe injuries).

Tendon Injuries and Disorders

The three main types of tendon injuries and disorders are: Tendinitis and ruptured tendons, Osgood-Schlatter disease, and Iliotibial band syndrome.

Tendon injuries range from tendinitis (inflammation of a tendon) to a ruptured (torn) tendon. Torn tendons most often occur from: Overusing a tendon (particularly in some sports); the tendon stretches like a worn-out rubber band and becomes inflamed, and trying to break a fall. If thigh muscles contract, the tendon can tear. This is most likely to happen in older people with weak tendons.

One type of tendinitis of the knee is called jumper's knee. In sports that require jumping, such as basketball, the tendon can become inflamed or can tear.

Osgood-Schlatter disease is caused by stress or tension on part of the growth area of the upper shin bone. It causes swelling in the knee and upper part of the shin bone. It can happen if a person's tendon tears away from the bone, taking a piece of bone with it. Young people who run and jump while playing sports can have this type of injury.

Iliotibial band syndrome occurs when a tendon rubs over the outer bone of the knee causing swelling. It happens if the knee is overused for a long time. This sometimes occurs in sports training.

Treatment for tendon injuries and disorders includes: Rest, ice, elevation, anti-inflammatory remedies such as bromelain, boswellia, or ginger to relieve pain and reduce swelling, limiting sports activity, exercise for stretching and strengthening, a cast, if there is a partial tear, or possibly surgery for complete tears or very severe injuries.

How Can People Prevent Knee Problems?

Some knee problems (such as those resulting from an accident) can't be prevented. But many knee problems can be prevented by doing the following:

- Warm up before playing sports. Walking and stretching are good warm-up exercises. Stretching the muscles in the front and the back of the thighs is a good way to warm up the knees.

- Make the leg muscles strong by doing certain exercises (for example, walking up stairs, riding a stationary bicycle, or working out with weights).

- Avoid sudden changes in the intensity of exercise.

- Increase the force or duration of activity slowly.

- Wear shoes that fit and are in good condition.

- Maintain a healthy weight. Extra weight puts pressure on the knees.

What Types of Exercise Are Best for Someone With Knee Problems?

Three types of exercise are best for people with arthritis:
Range-of-motion exercises. These exercises help maintain or increase flexibility. They also help relieve stiffness in the knee.
Strengthening exercises: These exercises help maintain or increase muscle strength. Strong muscles help support and protect joints with arthritis.
Aerobic or endurance exercises. These exercises improve heart function and blood circulation. They also help control weight. Some studies show that aerobic exercise can reduce swelling in some joints.

Treating Knee Problems in a Nutshell

- Treat knee injuries with RICE (Rest/Ice/Compression/Elevation).
- Have the injury assessed by a healthcare professional.
- When applicable begin use of anti-inflammatory products such as: Bromelain, Ginger, Boswella, Turmeric, etc...
- Let pain be your guide as to the amount and type of exertion you place on the injured knee.
- Work around the injured area if it does not cause pain.
- When inflammation has subsided you can heat the area prior to performing beneficial movements.
- Consider acupuncture as a viable means of treatment.

- Massage performed by a knowledgeable practitioner can be helpful.
- Take Pharmaceutical Grade Fish Oil: 2 -6 grams per day (depending on your weight).
- Make sure you are getting adequate nutrition in the form of proper diet (previously discussed) and supplementation.
- In all joint problems be sure you are getting an adequate amount of fresh and pure water on a daily basis.

Shoulder Problems

The most movable joint in the body, the shoulder is also one of the most potentially unstable joints. As a result, it is the site of many common problems. They include sprains, strains, dislocations, separations, tendonitis, bursitis, torn rotator cuffs, frozen shoulder, fractures, and arthritis. Anyone who has worked out with weights or played in various sports has probably had some sort of a shoulder injury in his or her history.

According to the Centers for Disease Control and Prevention, almost fourteen million people in the United States sought medical care in 2003 for shoulder problems.

Let's take a closer look at the shoulder joint. The shoulder joint is composed of three bones: the clavicle (collarbone), the scapula (shoulder blade), and the humerus (upper arm bone). Two joints facilitate movement of the shoulder. The acromioclavicular (ah-KRO-me-o-klah-VIK-u-lahr; AC) joint is located between the acromion (ah-KRO-me-on; part of the scapula that forms the highest point of the shoulder) and the clavicle. The glenohumeral joint, commonly called the shoulder joint, is a ball-and-socket-type joint that helps move the shoulder forward and backward and allows the arm to rotate in a circular fashion or hinge out and up away from the body. (The "ball," or humerus, is the top, rounded portion of the upper arm bone; the "socket," or glenoid, is a dish-shaped part of the outer edge of the scapula into which the ball fits.) The capsule is a soft tissue envelope that encircles the glenohumeral joint, and a thin, smooth synovial membrane lines it.

The shoulder joint can be compared to a golf ball and tee, in which the ball can easily slip off the flat tee. Because the bones provide little inherent stability to the shoulder joint, it is highly dependent on surrounding soft tissues such as capsule ligaments and the muscles surrounding the rotator cuff to hold the ball in place. The shoulder is relatively unstable but highly mobile, allowing an individual to place the hand in numerous positions. It is in fact, one of the most mobile joints in the human body.

The bones of the shoulder are held in place by muscles, tendons, and ligaments. Tendons are tough cords of tissue that attach the shoulder muscles to bone and assist the muscles in moving the shoulder. Ligaments attach shoulder bones to each other, providing stability. For example, three glenohumeral ligaments anchor the front of the joint capsule. The rotator cuff is a structure composed of tendons that work along with associated muscles to hold the ball at the top of the humerus in the glenoid socket and provide mobility and strength to the shoulder joint. It contains two filmy sac-like structures called bursa which permit smooth gliding between bones, muscles, and tendons. They cushion and protect the rotator cuff from the bony arch of the acromion. [31]

The shoulder is easily injured because the ball of the upper arm is larger than the shoulder socket that holds it. To remain stable, its muscles, tendons, and ligaments must anchor the shoulder.

Although the shoulder is easily injured during sporting activities and manual labor, the primary source of shoulder problems appears to be the natural age-related degeneration of the surrounding soft tissues such as those found in the rotator cuff. The incidence of rotator cuff problems rises dramatically as a function of age and is generally seen among individuals who are more than sixty years old. Often, the dominant and non-dominant arm will be affected to a similar degree. Overuse of the shoulder can lead to more rapid age-related deterioration.

Rotator Cuff Disease: Tendonitis and Bursitis

These conditions are closely related and may occur alone or in combination.

---

[31] www.niams.nih.gov/hi/topics/shoulderprobs, National Institute of Arthritis and Musculoskelatal and Skin Diseases.

Tendonitis is inflammation (redness, soreness, and swelling) of a tendon. In tendonitis of the shoulder, the rotator cuff and/or biceps tendon become inflamed, usually as a result of being pinched by surrounding structures. The injury may vary from mild inflammation to involvement of most of the rotator cuff. When the rotator cuff tendon becomes inflamed and thickened, it may get trapped under the acromion. Squeezing of the rotator cuff is called impingement syndrome.

Bursitis, or inflammation of the bursa sacs that protect the shoulder, may accompany tendonitis and impingement syndrome. Inflammation caused by a disease such as rheumatoid arthritis may cause rotator cuff tendonitis and bursitis. Sports involving overuse of the shoulder and occupations requiring frequent overhead reaching are other potential causes of irritation to the rotator cuff or bursa and may lead to inflammation and impingement.

If the rotator cuff and bursa are irritated, inflamed, and swollen, they may become squeezed between the head of the humerus and the acromion. Repeated motion involving the arms, or the effects of the aging process on shoulder movement over many years, may also irritate and wear down the tendons, muscles, and surrounding structures.

Signs and Symptoms: Signs of these conditions include the slow onset of discomfort and pain in the upper shoulder or upper third of the arm and/or difficulty sleeping on the shoulder. Tendonitis and bursitis also cause pain when the arm is lifted away from the body or overhead. If tendonitis involves the biceps tendon (the tendon located in front of the shoulder that helps bend the elbow and turn the forearm), pain will occur in the front or side of the shoulder and may travel down to the elbow and forearm. Pain may also occur when the arm is forcefully pushed upward overhead.

A diagnosis of tendonitis and bursitis begins with a medical history and physical examination. X rays do not show tendons or the bursa, but may be helpful in ruling out bony abnormalities or arthritis. The doctor may remove and test fluid from the inflamed area to rule out infection.

Treatment: The first step in treating these conditions is to reduce pain and inflammation with rest, ice, and natural anti-inflammatory herbs or enzymes. In some cases, the doctor or therapist will use ultrasound (gentle sound-wave vibrations) to warm deep tissues and improve blood flow. Gentle stretching and strengthening exercises are added gradually. These may be preceded or followed by use of an ice pack. If there is no improvement, the doctor may want to inject a corticosteroid medicine into the space under the acromion. While steroid injections are a common treatment, they must be used with extreme caution, and in my opinion as a last resort, because they may lead to tendon rupture. At this point I would recommend that you find a good acupuncturist and let him try to assist the shoulder in the healing process.

Many years ago I tore a tendon in the rotator cuff area and I had acupuncture done to the area for three months, and it healed quite well. Traditional medical doctors wanted to perform surgery, but I was glad that I had the knowledge and forethought to avoid that surgery and pursue less invasive treatments.

If there is still no improvement after six to twelve months, the doctor may recommend either arthroscopic or open surgery to repair damage and relieve pressure on the tendons and bursa sac. Surgery should always be a last resort effort in my opinion!

Rotator cuff tendons often become inflamed from overuse, aging, or a fall on an outstretched hand or another traumatic cause. Sports or occupations requiring repetitive overhead motion or heavy lifting can also place a significant strain on rotator cuff muscles and tendons. Over time, as a function of aging, tendons become weaker and degenerate. Eventually, this degeneration can lead to complete tears of both muscles and tendons. These tears are surprisingly common. In fact, a tear of the rotator cuff is not necessarily an abnormal situation in older individuals if there is no significant pain

215

or disability. Fortunately, these tears do not lead to any pain or disability in most people. However, some individuals can develop very significant pain as a result of these tears and they may require treatment.

Signs and Symptoms: Typically, a person with a rotator cuff injury feels pain over the deltoid muscle at the top and outer side of the shoulder, especially when the arm is raised or extended out from the side of the body. Motions like those involved in getting dressed can be painful. The shoulder may feel weak, especially when trying to lift the arm into a horizontal position. A person may also feel or hear a click or pop when the shoulder is moved. Pain or weakness on outward or inward rotation of the arm may indicate a tear in a rotator cuff tendon. The patient also feels pain when lowering the arm to the side after the shoulder is moved backward and the arm is raised.

A doctor may detect weakness but may not be able to determine from a physical examination where the tear is located. X rays, if taken, may appear normal. An MRI or ultrascund can help detect a full tendon tear or a partial tendon tear.

It is recommended that patients with a rotator cuff injury rest the shoulder, apply heat or cold to the sore area, and take a natural anti-inflammatory product such as bromelain, ginger, boswella or turmeric. Other treatments might be added, such as electrical stimulation of muscles and nerves, ultrasound, magnet therapy, or acupuncture. Exercises could be added to the treatment program to build flexibility and strength and restore the shoulder's function. If there is no improvement with these conservative treatments and functional impairment persists, the doctor may want to perform arthroscopic or open surgical repair of the torn rotator cuff.

Treatment for rotator cuff disease usually depends on the severity of the injury, the age and health status of the patient and the length of time a given patient may have had the condition. Patients with rotator cuff tendonitis or bursitis that does not include a complete tear of the tendon can usually be treated without surgery. Nonsurgical treatments include the use of anti-inflammatory products, followed by rehabilitative rotator cuff strengthening exercises. These treatments are best undertaken with the guidance of a health-care professional such as a physical therapist, who works in conjunction with the treating physician.

Generally speaking, individuals who are older and have had shoulder pain for a longer period of time can be treated with non-operative measures even in the presence of a complete rotator cuff tear. These people are often treated similarly to those who have pain, but do not have a rotator cuff tear. Again, anti-inflammatory products, acupuncture, magnet therapy, and rehabilitative exercises can be very effective.

Arthritis of the shoulder is a degenerative disease caused by either wear and tear of the cartilage (osteoarthritis) or an inflammation (rheumatoid arthritis) of one or more joints. Arthritis not only affects joints, but may also affect supporting structures such as muscles, tendons, and ligaments.

Signs and symptoms: The usual signs of arthritis of the shoulder are pain, particularly over the acromioclavicular joint, and a decrease in shoulder motion.

A doctor may suspect the patient has arthritis when there is both pain and swelling in the joint. The diagnosis may be confirmed by a physical examination and X rays. Blood tests may be helpful for diagnosing rheumatoid arthritis, but other tests may be needed as well. Analysis of synovial fluid from the shoulder joint may be helpful in diagnosing some kinds of arthritis.

Treatment of shoulder arthritis depends in part on the type of arthritis. Osteoarthritis of the shoulder could treated with anti-inflammatory products, such as those mentioned previously. Rheumatoid arthritis may require physical therapy and additional anti-inflammatory products and fish oil that is high in omega three fatty acids.

Treating Shoulder Problems in a Nutshell

- Treat Shoulder Injuries with RICE .(Rest/Ice/Compression/Elevation).
- Have the injury assessed by a healthcare professional.
- When applicable begin use of anti-inflammatory products such as: Bromelain, Ginger, Boswella, Turmeric, etc...
- Let pain be your guide when trying to exercise the injured area.
- Work around the injured area if it does not cause pain.
- When inflammation has subsided you can heat the area prior to performing beneficial movements.
- Consider acupuncture as a viable means of treatment.
- Massage performed by a knowledgeable practitioner can be helpful.
- Take Pharmaceutical Grade Fish Oil: 2 -6 grams per day (depending on your weight).
- Make sure you are getting adequate nutrition in the form of proper eating (previously discussed) and supplementation.
- As in all joint problems you should be certain you are getting an adequate amount of fresh and pure water.

High Blood Pressure

Do you have high blood pressure? Some people never even get it checked, and they run the many risk factors associated with this disease. First, we need to establish what the categories of blood pressure ratings are:

- *Borderline Hypertension: 120 – 160/90 – 94*
- *Mild Hypertension: 140 – 160/95 – 104*
- *Moderate Hypertension: 140 – 180/105 – 114*
- *Severe Hypertension: 160+/115+*

Your first task if you have never checked your blood pressure is to get it checked. Many pharmacies, such as Walmart or Walgreen's have machines to check your blood pressure for free. So, there is no excuse! A word of caution for those of you that have large arms; some of these machines are made to accommodate up to thirteen inch upper arms only! Another word of caution is to be aware of "White coat syndrome." White coat syndrome is the raise in blood pressure due to the presence of a person (i.e. doctor, nurse, or lab tech) wearing a white lab coat or the presence of one of these people without the lab jacket. It is best to take your blood pressure in a relaxed setting such as your own home.

This can be accomplished by purchasing a blood pressure device from your local pharmacy or department store. A digital device is usually the easiest one to use.

Approximately eighty percent of people with high blood pressure fall in the borderline to moderate range. These cases can usually be brought under control with dietary changes and lifestyle changes, such as adding exercise to your daily regime.

In ninety to ninety-five percent of cases, scientists do not know what causes high blood pressure. They have identified some factors that contribute to higher blood pressure. These are arteriosclerosis (or hardening of the arteries), thickening or hypertrophy of the artery wall, and excess contraction of the arterioles (small arteries).

Blood pressure is the force in the arteries when the heart beats (systolic pressure) and when the heart is at rest (diastolic pressure). It's measured in millimeters of mercury (mm Hg). High blood pressure directly increases the risk of coronary heart disease (which leads to heart attack) and stroke, especially when it's present with other risk factors.

Hypertension is known as the "silent killer" because in many cases there are no symptoms until serious complications develop. People with very high blood pressure can experience pulsating headaches (especially in the morning), visual disturbances, nausea and vomiting. Untreated high blood pressure can damage heart, kidneys and eyes leading to angina, heart attack, heart failure, kidney failure, peripheral vascular disease, retinopathy, stroke and abnormal heart beat.

Complications of high blood pressure include heart attack, congestive heart failure, arteriosclerosis, aortic dissection, kidney disease, stroke, brain damage, and vision problems.

Your lifestyle, if adjusted as outlined in this book, can have an enormous affect on your blood pressure and cardiovascular health in general. If you are overweight, every ten pound reduction can lower blood-pressure by five to twenty points. Reducing sodium intake for salt sensitive people was shown to reduce blood pressure two to eight points. Limiting your alcohol consumption to two glasses for men and one glass for women (and light weighted individuals) can lower blood-pressure by two to four points. Cutting caffeine can also make a difference.

In traditional Chinese medicine, high blood pressure is often viewed as a problem of circulation of energy (qi) in the body. Poor diet and emotional imbalance are just some of the factors that can lead to this condition. A combination of acupuncture and herbs is often recommended to balance energy flow. Secondary high blood pressure is often due to exhaustion of energy reserves. This is called kidney yin deficiency. The treatment goal is to build up and restore energy.

Treating High Blood Pressure in a Nutshell

- Get light to moderate exercise on a regular basis, and try to maintain a proper body weight for your structure.
- Practice stress reducing activities (i.e. yoga, tai chi, meditation, prayer, and get an adequate amount of sleep).
- Eat a high fiber diet (i.e. non-instant oats, brown rice, buckwheat and millet are a few high fiber foods you can include in your diet).
- Eat plenty of fruits and vegetables.
- Eat fresh garlic if feasible or in capsule form otherwise.
- Restrict sodium intake.
- Avoid all alcohol, tobacco and caffeine products.
- Limit animal fats.
- Supplement with calcium (1,500 – 3,000 mg. daily); and magnesium (750 – 1,000 mg. daily).
- Omega 3 Fish Oil: 2 – 6 grams per day.
- Flax Seed Oil: 2 grams per day.
- Take a good whole food multi vitamin/mineral supplement daily.
- Take Hawthorn as directed on the bottle daily.

Type II Diabetes

Let's take a quick course on diabetes, in general, so that you will have a greater understanding of the material forthcoming.

Insulin, which is a hormone produced by the pancreas, regulates the amount of glucose in your blood. Normally, your body's cells are impermeable (cannot be penetrated) to glucose. However, in the presence of insulin, specific cell receptors are activated and glucose is allowed to rapidly enter the cell. Once inside muscle and fat cells, glucose can be utilized for energy.

The amount of glucose circulating is tightly regulated by the body by releasing insulin. When glucose levels exceed a certain point, the pancreas secretes more insulin into the blood to help move the glucose out of the blood and into your cells. When blood glucose levels get too low, the body releases glucose from stores kept in the liver and this triggers you to eat.

Problems arise when the pancreas does not produce insulin, or when the pancreas produces very little insulin or when the body is unable to utilize the insulin in a normal manner due to "insulin resistance."

Without the insulin, glucose remains in the blood and reaches levels that are toxic. In addition, because the glucose remains in the blood, key organs are deprived of the necessary fuel to function. There are basically three types of diabetes:

- *Type I Diabetics* have a severe deficiency of insulin and comprise approximately ten percent of total cases. Type I Diabetes is typically diagnosed in childhood and is sometimes called juvenile-onset diabetes mellitus. Type I Diabetes can also occur in older people who, for some reason, lose their pancreatic beta cells. Common causes include alcohol, pathology, surgery, etc. Type I Diabetics require daily insulin to survive; hence they are sometimes called insulin-dependent diabetics.

- *Type II Diabetics* produce insulin but the body is unable to utilize this insulin (insulin resistance). Ninety percent of diabetics have Type II Diabetes. Type II Diabetes can be controlled with diet, exercise, weight loss and medications. Because this type of diabetes affects the most people in the fifty plus group, we will concentrate our information on preventing and treating it.

- *Gestational Diabetes* (Pregnancy) develops during the second and third trimesters of pregnancy. Gestational diabetes typically goes away after delivery. Women with gestational diabetes are likely to develop it again during subsequent pregnancies. These women are also susceptible to Type II Diabetes later in life. Babies born of diabetic mothers are often larger than normal.

Type II Diabetes, also known as adult onset diabetes or non-insulin - dependent diabetes is responsible for about 70,000 deaths annually, and was the seventh ranking cause of death in 1999. About 95% of the people who have diabetes have this type.[32] This form of diabetes tends to occur in people who are older than forty-five and overweight. The number of persons diagnosed with this disease in the United States has grown steadily and rapidly over the years. In 1958 there were approximately 1.5 million cases and in 1997 there were 10.3 million. It is important to remember that this disease also makes a person at risk for other diseases such as heart attacks and stroke; and is the leading cause of new cases of blindness, fatal kidney disease, and lower extremity amputations.[33]

Type II Diabetes is a disease that occurs when the cells of the body become resistant to insulin. The reason cells become resistant to insulin is because these cells have been bombarded with an overproduction of insulin for many years. The human body will

---

[32] www.cdc.gov/nchs/fastats.htm/Deaths/Mortality, National Center for Human Statistics, 11/04/01.
[33] www.cdc.gov/nccdphp/diabetes.htm/ ,Diabetes, National Center for Chronic Disease Prevention and Health Promotion, 11/03/01.

produce insulin when we consume carbohydrates; that is, sugars and starches that are broken down into sugars.

When a diet consists of too many simple carbohydrates, insulin is produced in large amounts. The simple carbohydrates that are the culprits in this case are foods that contain white sugar, white flour, or white rice products. So, you say to yourself, why not eliminate these foods from the diet? Excellent deduction!

In my opinion Type II Diabetes is totally treatable with dietary changes and an exercise regime. If we were to eliminate the white sugar, white flour, and white rice products from our diet we will be on the right path.

Preventing Type II Diabetes in a Nutshell

- Eliminate white sugar, white flour, and white rice products from the diet.
- Eat only unrefined carbohydrates (whole grains or sprouted products).
- Exercise daily.
- Avoid all tobacco products, and minimize alcohol consumption.
- Include plenty of raw fruits and vegetables, berries, brewers yeast, dairy products, egg yolks, fish, garlic, kelp, sauerkraut, soybeans, and cinnamon in your diet.
- Try to balance each meal in regard to the protein and carbohydrate content.
- Take a good whole food multi-vitamin/mineral supplement daily.
- Include alpha lipoic acid (100 – 200 mg. daily) as a supplement.

Treating Type II Diabetes

- Do all of the above plus the following:
- Take Chromium Picolinate: 400 – 600 mcg. daily.

- Garlic: fresh or as a capsule taken as directed daily.
- Extra B-Complex: daily as directed.
- Co Q10: 100 mg. daily.
- Spirulina: daily as directed.

Heart Health

Why do you need to keep a healthy heart? Heart disease is the number one cause of death in men and women; greater than the next five causes of death combined! According to the latest estimates by the American Heart Association, over sixty-four million Americans have one or more forms of cardiovascular disease. Fortunately, there are ways to significantly lower your chances of developing heart disease and reverse the effects of a current heart condition you may or may not be aware of.

Some of the indicators for possible heart disease are cholesterol buildup in the form of arterial plaque, high levels of triglycerides, high levels of homocysteine, obesity, family history that is repeated mainly by having the same lifestyle of one's parents, cigarette smoking, large alcohol consumption, lack of exercise, and poor nutritional habits.

What is cholesterol and is it all bad?

Cholesterol is a necessary component for your body's health. It is essentially a non-soluble waxy substance that your body uses to make hormones, cell walls and nerve sheaths. There is good cholesterol and there is bad cholesterol, as discussed below.

What's the difference between LDL cholesterol and HDL cholesterol?
LDL cholesterol (low density lipoprotein) is the bad or oxidized form. LDL cholesterol attaches itself to artery walls, creating plaque that can build up and eventually block your arteries, which could result in a heart attack or stroke. There are large and small bubble LDL, and it has been found that the large bubble LDL is not harmful. Knowing this, you should want your small bubble LDL cholesterol levels to be as low as possible.

HDL cholesterol (high density lipoprotein) is the good form. HDL cholesterol travels around in your bloodstream, picks up excess LDL cholesterol and brings it back to your liver to be reprocessed. Therefore, HDL cholesterol is cleaning out your body. You want your HDL cholesterol levels to be as high as possible.

What is the ideal HDL/LDL ratio in the bloodstream? Your total cholesterol is an important figure, but even more important is the ratio of LDL (bad) cholesterol to HDL (good) cholesterol. Following are the normal and optimal levels of cholesterol levels.

Total Cholesterol – Levels up to 199 mg/dL

Optimal Levels: Between 180-220 mg/dL

LDL Cholesterol - Normal Levels: up to 129 mg/dL
Optimal Levels: Under 100 mg/dL

HDL Cholesterol - Normal Levels: no lower than 35mg/dL
Optimal Levels: Over 50 mg/dL

Summary: For optimal health, you should keep your LDL chole-sterol down and keep your HDL cholesterol up! If you follow the nutritional guidelines presented in this book you are likely to achieve the proper ratio of HDL/LDL.

Taking a special natural cholesterol lowering formula with vitamins, minerals and herbal extracts to help lower LDL cholesterol levels as well as decrease triglycerides (fats) will help to promote overall heart health.

The relationship between increased homocysteine and heart disease is well established in the medical community. Yet unlike the other three predictors of heart disease, i.e. cholesterol, triglycerides and C

Reactive Protein, homocysteine levels are influenced by what you DON'T eat rather than what you do eat.

Approximately 10% of coronary deaths can be attributed to high levels of homocysteine in the blood.

What is homocysteine?
Homocysteine is an abnormal protein that is created when a specific amino acid called methionine is metabolized. In most people homocysteine is quickly cleared out of the arteries and therefore does not create a problem. However, for some people homocysteine is not efficiently cleared out and can pose significant health risks.

What causes elevated homocysteine levels in the blood?
Studies have shown that high levels of homocysteine are caused by a lack of nutrients in the diet, particularly the B group of vitamins. Without these essential vitamins your body is unable to produce the enzymes necessary to remove homocysteine efficiently from your blood. Homocysteine will cause damage to your arteries when present in high concentrations - hence the link between homocysteine and heart disease.

How can you treat homocysteine and lower your risk?
A lack of B Vitamins leads to elevated homocysteine levels which is why high homocysteine and vegetarian diets are directly related. Fortunately the situation is easily treatable. In the late 1960s Dr. Kilmer McCully determined through extensive research that by taking adequate amounts of folic acid, along with vitamins B6 and B12, your levels of homocysteine will normalize.

Preventing Heart Problems in a Nutshell

- Exercise daily, and perform cardiovascular exercise as discussed previously at minimum of four times per week for twenty minutes or more.

- Eat a healthy diet as previously outlined in this book.
  A. Eliminate intake of trans fats and hydrogenated oils found in margarine, fast food, fried food, etc.
  B. Eliminate refined sugar intake.
  C. Use extra virgin olive oil and garlic in cooking.
  D. Add Omega 3 Fatty Acids to your diet - the best source is Fish Oil.
- If your cholesterol is high, you can lower cholesterol naturally with policosanol, guggulipid and other herbal extracts as well as Fish Oil. Remember, only a small portion of your cholesterol comes from what you eat; the majority is manufactured by your liver when you consume refined carbohydrates (white sugar, white flour or white rice).
- If your triglyceride levels are too high, lower your refined carbohydrate intake. Fish oil, Vitamin C, guggulipid and green tea are safe natural ways to lower triglyceride levels.
- Keep your weight within recommended limits - obesity is a leading cause of heart disease.
- Try to reduce stress and anxiety - they can lead to high blood pressure and other health conditions.
- Do not smoke, and if you do…QUIT before you have a major problem.
- Do not drink, or drink in moderation if you must.

Menopause

Included in the physical change for middle aged women is *menopause*. Women are born with several hundred thousand ova, which begin to mature at puberty. Around three to four hundred cycles later, ovulation becomes erratic and finally stops. Menopause is considered to have occurred when a whole year has passed without menstruation. At this time, ovarian estrogen production occurs for a while but eventually will cease. Deprived of the stimulatory effects of estrogen, the reproductive organs and breasts begin to atrophy. The possible symptoms of menopause are: headaches, dizziness, joint pain, hot flashes, loss of bone mass, and slowly rising blood cholesterol levels.

I must inform the reader at this time that most women living in third world countries do not go through the customary symptoms that are experienced in industrialized nations. Some of the reasons for this are due to diet, amount of physical exertion, and expectation of what menopause is going to be like. I've mentioned expectation theory earlier in this book, but this is another example of how a person's expectations are usually met. Unfortunately, this works to our detriment at times.

Low dose estrogen therapy is often encouraged by medical doctors for women at this time. Premarin and Provera are prescribed to many women, but the risks of certain cancers and heart attacks are overlooked. One of the reasons doctors prescribe estrogen replacement is due to the connection between loss of estrogen and osteoporosis. Bones become fragile and more likely to break. An alternative to Hormone-Replacement Therapy (HRT) is bio-identical hormone replacement therapy, exercise, and a proper diet.

Besides HRT, diet and exercise have been associated with better experiences of menopause and its symptoms. Sometimes a lifestyle change needs to be considered. There's a stress connection and a lifestyle connection. In one study (*Prevention Magazine, Aug...1994 vol.46 pg .84))*, the more stress a woman reported in her life, the more symptoms she had. Fifty-five percent in the high-stress group reported suffering from six or more symptoms as compared to just twenty percent in the low-stress group. It is unclear whether more stress contributes to menopause symptoms or more symptoms contribute to stress. It has been reported that exercising helps to relieve the symptoms. Researchers at Tufts University report that weight training helps to slow bone loss, another symptom of menopause. Exercise has also been associated with a better experience of menopause.

The conventional use of synthetic hormone replacement therapy was studied by the women's Health Initiative and then canceled due to the high risk of breast cancer, heart disease, and stroke associated with the use of synthetic HRT (Premarin and Provera or PremPro). Sixteen thousand women, age fifty to seventy nine, were studied, and after five years it was found that women using this type of HRT had a twenty nine percent higher risk of breast cancer, a twenty six percent higher risk of heart disease, and a forty one percent higher risk of stroke. Typical side effects from these drugs include weight gain, fatigue, depression, irritability, headaches, insomnia, bloating, low thyroid function, low libido, gallbladder disease, and blood clots.

Dealing with Menopause in a Nutshell

- Eat a balanced diet as outlined in this book; limiting or totally eliminating refined carbohydrates is extremely helpful in dealing with female hormone problems in general.
- Remember, menopause is not a disease or disorder! It is a transition period in a woman's life.
- Avoid alcohol, caffeine, spicy foods, hot soups and drinks because they can trigger hot flashes, aggravate urinary problems, and cause mood swings to be more pronounced.
- Try some of these in combination or alone to relieve unpleasant symptoms of menopause: Black Cohosh,

Dong Quai, Vitamin E, Anise, Fennel, Licorice (for seven days or less at a time, or avoid if you have high blood pressure), Gotu Kola, Sarsaparilla, Squawvine, Unicorn Root, or Wild Yam.

- Exercise regularly as outlined in this book.
- Avoid the use of any synthetic hormone and use natural hormone replacement therapy when applicable.
- Use a saliva test to determine if you need to replace any hormones. Fat cells also produce estrogen in small amounts, so do not assume that you necessarily need more estrogen.
- Always replace hormones at a dosage that your body would produce naturally under good conditions.

Prostate Health

Prostate health is an issue that concerns most men over the age of fifty. Multiple studies show that prostate cancer can be prevented with proper diet and supplements. It has shown that dietary changes can have a favorable impact on this disease, even after diagnosis.[34] Perhaps you have no problems or symptoms of a problem, but never-the- less, it still remains a major concern for many men. So let's take a closer look at what this problem is all about.

In men, urine flows from the bladder through the urethra. BPH is a benign (noncancerous) enlargement of the prostate that blocks the flow of urine through the urethra. The prostate cells gradually multiply, creating an enlargement that puts pressure on the urethra; the "chute" through which urine and semen exit the body.

As the urethra narrows, the bladder has to contract more forcefully to push urine through the body. Over time, the bladder muscle may gradually become stronger, thicker, and overly sensitive; it begins to contract even when it contains small amounts of urine, causing a need to urinate frequently. Eventually, the bladder muscle cannot overcome the effect of the narrowed urethra, so urine remains in the bladder and it is not completely emptied.

Symptoms of an enlarged prostate can include:

- A weak or slow urinary stream
- A feeling of incomplete bladder emptying
- Difficulty starting urination
- Frequent urination
- Urgency to urinate
- Getting up frequently at night to urinate
- A urinary stream that starts and stops
- Straining to urinate

---

[34] Ornish, D et al: Intensive lifestyle changes may affect the progression of prostate cancer. J Urol Vol. 174:1065, 2005

When the bladder does not empty completely, you become at risk for developing urinary tract infections. Other serious problems can also develop over time, including bladder stones, blood in the urine, incontinence, and acute urinary retention (an inability to urinate). A sudden and complete inability to urinate is a medical emergency; you should see your doctor immediately. In rare cases, bladder and/or kidney damage can develop from BPH.

Most men put up with these problems for months, even years, before seeing a doctor. It generally isn't until they're getting up several times a night, and have trouble falling asleep again when they come in and seek medical attention.

Prostate growth and the trouble it causes vary greatly from person to person. Some people have more growth than others. Some people with very large prostates don't have trouble with voiding. It's a very individual thing.

The driving force in treatment is whether the symptoms are affecting your quality of life and whether a blockage is causing serious complications, such as inability to urinate, blood in the urine, bladder stones, kidney failure, or other bladder problems.

A few questions to ask yourself:

- How severe are your symptoms?
- Do symptoms prevent you from doing things you enjoy?
- Do they seriously affect your quality of life?
- Are they getting worse?
- Are you ready to accept some small risks to get rid of your symptoms?
- Do you know the risks associated with each treatment?
- Is it time to do something?

In the United States, prostate cancer is reaching epidemic proportions. One in six men will eventually be diagnosed, which translates to 220,000 new initiates every year.[35] Most of these prostate cancers will not be life threatening. Nevertheless, no man wants to hear that he has prostate cancer. So what can men do to prevent this disease?

They need to look at what they eat. Prostate cancer is primarily a disease of the overfed. We know this is true simply by comparing the outcomes in men on Asian diets with those eating a Western diet. Prostate cancer is just as common in the Orient as it is in the United States. However, the mortality rate in Asia is 20 times lower. Genetic differences cannot explain this because as soon as Asians move to the United States, their mortality rates start to approach those of other Americans.

As a general rule, men on the Asian continent eat a diet containing far lower amounts of animal protein than what's consumed in the Western world. In his recent book, *The China Study* (Benbella Books), Colin Campbell studied and compared the impact of low and high animal protein diets on the incidence and mortality of a variety of cancers, including prostate cancer. Campbell's book, while implicating excess protein in the diet, acknowledges the possibility that it may not be protein per se that's increasing cancer rates, but rather the fats that are associated with animal protein.

Campbell's observations are supported by various studies performed in the United States. These studies show that being overweight and overeating lead to an increased incidence of prostate cancer or increased aggressiveness of the disease.[36]-[37]-[38] Therefore, counseling

---

[35] A, et al: Cancer Statistics, 2006. Ca Cancer J Clin Vol. 56: 106-30, 2006

[36] Hsieh, Lillian et al: Association of energy intake with prostate cancer in a long-term aging study: Baltimore longitudinal study of aging (United States). Urology Vol. 61:297, 2003.

[37] Freedland, Stephen et al: Obesity and risk of biochemical progression following radical prostatectomy at a tertiary care referral center. The Journal of Urology Vol. 174:919, 2005.

[38] Amling, Christopher et al: Pathologic variables and recurrence rates as related to obesity and race in men with prostate cancer undergoing radical prostatectomy. Journal of Clinical Oncology Vol. 22:439, 2004

our patients about proper dietary practices, preventive supplements, pharmaceuticals when necessary, and knowledge of the dangers of indiscriminate eating should help reduce the incidence of prostate cancer.

Preventing Prostate Problems in a Nutshell

- Eat a whole food diet consisting of whole grains, raw nuts and seeds, unpolished brown rice, cruciferous vegetables (broccoli, Brussels sprouts, cabbage and cauliflower), spinach, yellow and deep orange vegetables (carrots, pumpkin, squash and yams), apples, cantaloupe, grapefruit, watermelon, tomatoes, tomato products, berries, brazil nuts, sunflower seeds, pumpkin seeds, cherries, grapes, mushrooms (shiitake, maitake, reishi, and cordyceps), garlic, and lentils.
- Drink freshly made vegetable and fruit juices (carrot and cabbage) daily.
- Exclude alcohol, coffee, and refined carbohydrates (white sugar, white flour, or white rice).
- Be sure to include Omega 3 fatty acids: in food such as salmon, sardines, mackerel, herring, or in supplement form (i.e. pharmaceutical grade fish oil: 2 – 6 grams per day; flax seed oil: 2 grams per day).
- Take a Whole Food Multi-Vitamin/Mineral daily.
- Supplement Co Q10: 100 mg. daily.
- Selenium: 200 mcg. Daily.
- Hi-B Complex daily.
- Ester C: 1000 mg. – 10,000 mg. daily (under guidance of your physician).
- Maitake Extract: 4 grams – 8 grams daily.

Vision Problems

The eyes are two of the most complicated organs in the human body. They are a very important part of our day-to-day life and there are several conditions that can affect the eyes. We all have experienced at one time or another some type of eye problem, irritation, dryness, red eye, or some more serious conditions like cataract or blindness.

Although most of the times eye problems are localized or within the eye itself, sometimes the eyes reflect diseases elsewhere in the body; for example, blurred vision can be a sign of diabetes, yellow eyes can be a clue to hepatitis, or a remarked difference in the pupil's size can indicate that a tumor is developing somewhere in the body.

The eye is one of nature's great feats of engineering, with millions of working parts that let you focus up close, far away and in between, all in spectacular color and three dimensions.

Of course, all of this complexity also means that things can sometimes get out of whack. There is nearsightedness, in which you have trouble focusing on distant objects, and farsightedness, where you can't see close-up things well. Some people think their arms are just getting shorter because we can't seem to focus any closer than arms length. If this is your problem you can perform arm stretching exercises by hanging heavy weights from one or both hands. That extra few inches in arm length may be just what you need to see that menu or book! As we age it does become more difficult to focus on objects that are close, and this is part of the aging process. Some people experience it while others may not.

There is glaucoma, a buildup of fluid pressure that can damage your optic nerve, and cataracts, opaque lenses that fog your vision. Diabetes can cause detached retinas and other complications. And macular degeneration—the deterioration of the macula, the part of the eye that's responsible for distinguishing fine details—is the leading cause of blindness in people over age fifty. Some of these problems require glasses, some may need surgery to fix, and some are irreversible.

Let's take a closer look at some of the eye problems that we may encounter, and give you ideas about ways to avoid these unwanted encounters.

Cataracts are a clouding of the eye lens that causes blurred vision and inability to focus, and is progressive and painless. The cataract becomes thicker with time until it blinds the eye. This is the number one cause of blindness in the world.

The most common type of cataracts is senile cataracts, which means that it mainly affects people sixty five and older. This type of cataract is caused by free radicals that damage the lens. It has been shown that glutathione, copper, and manganese can help to retard the growth of cataracts

Glaucoma is a very serious disease that affects the optic nerve; the pressure inside the eye increases damaging the nerve and causing vision loss and blindness. People over sixty-five are at risk, and people with diabetes are at risk as well.

This condition produces no symptoms, therefore people who suffer glaucoma do not find out until it's very advanced. Glaucoma probably has many causes; some scientists claim it to be related to stress, poor nutrition, and high blood pressure; also collagen deficiency has been linked to glaucoma.

Macular Degeneration is a serious eye disease that can lead to blindness. A regular diet high in omega-3 polyunsaturated fat from fish appears to reduce the risk of both early and late age related macular degeneration (AMD), according to an Australian study published in the *Archives of Ophthalmology*.

Researchers reported a seventy percent reduction in the risk of developing AMD in study subjects who ate three or more portions of fish per week. However, lower weekly consumption was also beneficial with people who ate fish once per week seeing a forty percent reduction in risk.

When researchers calculated in terms of specific types of fats, they found that people with the lowest dietary intake of mono-unsaturated fatty acids and omega-3 poly-unsaturated fatty acids, especially alpha-linolenic acid, may be at a greater risk of developing AMD[39]

Another vision problem that may be experienced by people over fifty is our difficulty with our night vision. The average sixty year old person needs seven times as much light as a twenty year old to see well in the dark, according to the American Optometric Association. So brighten up the rooms of your home with sixty or one hundred watt neodymium light bulbs, suggests Bruce Rosenthal, O.D., chief of low-vision programs at Lighthouse International, a vision rehabilitation organization in New York City. These bulbs provide higher contrast and produce fewer glares than regular light bulbs, so you should be able to see better at night. Neodymium bulbs are available at specialty lighting stores and from some mail-order catalog companies.

There are many things you can do to ensure eye health for the duration of your life. Let's look at some of these concepts.

Drink less coffee, says Jay Cohen, O.D., associate professor at the State University of New York College of Optometry in New York City. "One study about ten years ago looked at caffeine and the effect it has on the focusing system of the eye, and it's a negative effect." Other sources of caffeine to avoid, according to Dr. Cohen, include tea, chocolate and cola as well as many pain relievers.

He also advises eating an overall healthy diet that relies more on fresh fruits and vegetables than on refined sugars and high-cholesterol animal products. "My feeling is you should have the best possible diet for the best possible vision," says Dr. Cohen. Foods

---

[39] http://video.swansonvitamins.com/e_files/ResearchUpdate/060603.

that are high in carotenes, such as broccoli, kale, cauliflower, peas, beets, green beans, Brussels sprouts and cabbage, are especially good.

A daily supplement that contains Vitamin E and Vitamin A are very helpful for vision problems associated with aging, such as farsightedness, says Jay Cohen, O.D., associate professor at the State University of New York College of Optometry in New York City. "Many studies show that people who take antioxidant vitamin supplements are at much lower risk of developing age-related changes in the eyes."

You can strengthen eye muscles and improve vision with a series of simple yoga exercises, writes yoga teacher Rosalind Widdowson in her book *The Joy of Yoga*. She suggests doing the entire sequence of exercises described below once a day in the order listed.

She says that you can do all of these exercises sitting in a straight-back chair, with your feet resting comfortably on the floor.

Distancing: Place your left hand in your lap and stretch your right arm straight out at eye level with your palm facing you. Then make a gentle fist, and raise your index finger. Look down at your nose with both eyes; then switch your glance to your raised finger. Then look as far into the distance as you can. Switch back to your finger, then your nose. Do this five times. Repeat this exercise with your left arm extended and your right hand in your lap.

Widdowson says you should also do a set of these exercises first with one eye closed, then with the other closed.

Verticals/horizontals: Sit with both hands in your lap. Hold your head straight up, looking forward. With both eyes, look right, then straight ahead, then left and then straight again. Repeat five times.

After this, look up, then straight, then down and then straight again. Repeat five times.

Diagonal: Again, sit with both hands in your lap and your head held straight up. Start by looking up and right. Then in one smooth motion, move your glance diagonally until you're looking down and left. Return to looking up and right. Do this five times, then switch, looking up and left, moving down and right and returning up and left. Repeat this five times.

Circles: Sit with both hands in your lap and your head facing forward. Make a full circle with your eyes in a clockwise direction. Do this five times, and then perform five circles counterclockwise.

Expansion: Close your eyes tightly, then open them wide, looking at an object far off in the distance. Do this ten times.

Preventing & Treating Vision Problems in a Nutshell

- A good whole food multi vitamin/mineral supplement should be taken daily. Find one that has lutein, zeaxanthin, and carotenoids as part of the formula.
- Extra Vitamin A (25,000 IU if you are not pregnant) taken daily.
- Free Form Amino Acid Complex daily.
- The amino acid Taurine daily.
- B-Complex daily.
- Vitamin C (1000mg) taken three to four times per day.
- Vitamin E (400 IU) daily.
- Bayberry bark, cayenne, and red raspberry can be beneficial.
- Bilberry extract may improve your regular vision and your night vision.
- Perform eye exercises regularly and perform other exercises mentioned in this book regularly.
- Eat a diet that includes plenty of fresh vegetables: broccoli, raw cabbage, carrots, cauliflower, green

vegetables, squash, seeds, nuts, and watercress; drink juice from vegetables.

- Eliminate white sugar, white flour and white rice from the diet.
- Drink plenty (apprx. 60 – 80 oz.) of fresh water every day.

Digestive Problems

At some point in our lives we all have had to deal with some type of digestive disorder. It may have been mild as in the case of eating a type of food that doesn't agree with us, or it may have been more severe, such as an ulcer or problem with one of the digestive organs.

As we age, the process takes a toll on the GI tract. Aging muscles, including the digestive muscles, contract more slowly, take plenty of time relaxing, and move their contents along at a more leisurely pace. For the most part, that in itself isn't going to cause any major problems — unless you become impatient, it takes drastic measures to hurry things along, or develop a condition that needs a doctor's attention. Many of the aging gastrointestinal system's failures can be prevented or corrected.

Let's take a closer look at each of these areas so that we all have a better understanding concerning our digestive system. The changes begin at the top, in the mouth, where the number of taste buds begins to decline with age, especially when we smoke, drink coffee, or use excessive amounts of salt, and spices on our food. As well as there is a reduced sensitivity of the taste buds that remains. The chewing muscles also begin to weaken. As a result, some older people lose interest in food, begin to lose weight, and develop nutritional deficiencies. Losing teeth may also reduce interest in eating. Good dental care is important to keep the teeth in shape so that eating doesn't become a problem. Brush your teeth often and floss them at least one time per day.

Swallowing can also become more difficult as people age. Such problems are usually the result of neurological or muscular disorders. The very old may experience a weakening of the muscles of the esophagus, which contract less vigorously around food after swallowing. Acid reflux is often a problem in the elderly, the result of the decline in esophageal contractions and in the function of the lower esophageal sphincter muscle. However, since the esophagus may be less sensitive to acid with age, acid reflux may not result in heartburn. Instead, patients may complain of nausea or vague chest discomfort. A doctor should evaluate any new onset of difficulty in swallowing because the problem could be related to cancer of the esophagus or to a motor disorder (achalasia), more common in those who are older.

As people age, the stomach continues to make acid, but in many middle aged people (fifty to one hundred years young), acid production declines because of years of carrying *Helicobacter pylori* infection in the stomach, leading to long-term gastritis and to a weakening of the stomach lining. While a reduction in gastric acid does not usually interfere with digestion, it can lead to two disorders that are common in the people as they age: vitamin B_{12} deficiency, which can result in anemia and nerve damage, and excessive bacterial growth in the small intestine, resulting in poor absorption of nutrients and poor digestion. These problems can be corrected with the proper intervention.

Moving one's bowels may be the most frequent gastrointestinal challenge associated with aging. The problem is usually the result of a poorly functioning or diseased large intestine. Problems with this organ can also result in diarrhea and hemorrhoids. In addition, the risk for colon cancer and polyps increases with age. In fact, one in three middle aged people (fifty to one hundred years young) have one or more polyps in the colon. That's why a screening exam called a colonoscopy is recommended on a regular basis after age fifty. Since colon cancer evolves from polyps, removal of polyps will keep colon cancer from getting started. In general, fewer stools are passed after one reaches the age of sixty five. In part, this may be the result of a change in diet to softer foods, a decreased appetite, or diminished muscular activity of the colon. Constipation may also be the result of a neurological problem.

The most important thing is to eat a balanced diet that includes plenty of fiber, unless your complaint is excess gas. Eat smaller meals and drink sufficient liquids. Eliminate caffeine (especially coffee), tobacco, and alcohol; and stay away from foods and medications that seem to upset your stomach.

It is a common cultural belief that one's emotions reside in your midsection. So it should be no surprise to learn that stress is a leading cause of many of these disorders, and reducing it can help you find relief not only from these gastrointestinal symptoms, but in many other ways as well. Try to relax more often and practice techniques that enhance relaxation. Simply practicing diaphragmic breathing on a regular basis can help to calm a person's mind and body.

Exercising on a regular basis can help your midsection in many ways. It will help it look better from the outside by reducing fat stores, and help it function better from the inside. Simply performing crunches (previously described in the section on abdominal exercises) on a daily basis can help move foods along the digestive system and help to keep a person's bowels move regularly.

Don't eat foods that disagree with you. We all know what most of them are, and unfortunately they are foods we usually enjoy, but we must remember the end result of eating them. When traveling, drink only bottled water and skip the street vendors. You'll cut down on your chances of getting traveler's diarrhea. Also, don't forget that ice comes from water. This was a hard learned lesson for my spouse on a recent trip to Africa.

The gastrointestinal tract does not operate independently. Problems in other parts of the body, including the mind, can have a profound impact on the gut. Live as healthy a lifestyle as possible, in body and mind alike. Though you may still need to consult a doctor from time to time, follow the approaches outlined in this book and you will increase your chances to live a disease free life.

Indigestion and nausea are generally caused by overeating, eating the wrong foods, combining foods that do not digest well together, stress, and ingesting harmful organisms.

To remedy indigestion or nausea you should chew your food thoroughly and minimize sweets and sugars of all kinds, and try to avoid combining foods that upset the digestive process. Using peppermint or chamomile tea, licorice root, anise or fennel seeds, tumeric, or aloe vera gel or juice with a touch of lemon can help with this problem as well. Some people benefit from a supplement of hydrochloric acid or bicarbonate at mealtime. Be sure to include healthy bacteria (probiotics) in capsule, powder, or liquid form.

If your condition persists after trying these remedies, you should ask your health care practitioner to test you for abnormal bacteria, yeast, or parasites.

Heartburn is caused by stress, eating while under stress, irritating foods such as caffeine, alcohol, strong spices, or infection by helicobacter pylori bacteria. This type of bacteria is a common cause of gastritis and ulcers.

To remedy this condition we must soothe and heal the upper intestinal membranes, reduce excess stomach acid, and eliminate any infection that may be present. We all have stomach acid, and it is actually the way our body protects us against bad bugs. However, in cases of heartburn, the delicate tissue at the stomach's entrance is being burned by the hydrochloric acid. Eating more alkaline vegetables (especially steamed vegetables) and their juices and broths can help calm the stomach.

Ingesting baking soda (one half of a teaspoon to one teaspoon) will directly counter stomach acid. A very effective treatment for heartburn or acid reflux is DGL (deglycyrrhizinated licorice). Simply chew one or two tablets once or twice a day between meals or for heartburn. Chamomile tea can also be helpful, as well as calcium or calcium/magnesium tablets or capsules, or buffered Vitamin C (calcium, magnesium, and/or potassium ascorbates).

For persistent heartburn that doesn't respond to dietary changes and natural remedies within a week or two, see your doctor for a possible solution, blood test for H. pylori, and a blood or stool test for parasites. If these don't reveal anything, you may need to see a gastroenterologist for a closer look at your stomach.

Constipation is usually caused by a lack of fluids or fiber in the diet, overeating, stress, low thyroid function, excess alcohol or caffeine, yeast overgrowth, and other harmful organisms. It involves slowing of the peristaltic activity of the intestines, and or a loss of tone in the abdominal muscles, which results in sluggish bowel function.

Some of the remedies for constipation are as simple as chewing your food well, drinking approximately sixty four ounces, or more, of pure water per day (should be accomplished between meals), or lemon water, or herbal tea. Be sure to get regular exercise and eat more salads, vegetables, and fruits. If you suspect yeast or harmful organisms, emphasize vegetables rather than fruit, due to the natural sweetness of the fruit, which can encourage yeast or bacterial overgrowth.

As for supplements, you can add more fiber, such as psyllium seed husks, as well as ground flax seeds and flaxseed oil. A magnesium supplement and/or increased levels of Vitamin C can help loosen the bowels. Probiotics may also help. On a temporary basis, you can use herbal tea laxatives such as aloe vera, cascara sagrada, senna leaf, fennel seeds, or other herbs. However, these remedies are best started on a weekend when you can stay at home and be close to the bathroom. Natural laxatives, such as cascara sagrada, can cause some cramping or an immediate need for a bowel movement at some undefined point after taking them. This can also occur with higher intake of magnesium.

Constipation may seem routine to many, but it is a concern that can lead to major health problems. When the body doesn't clear its waste materials on a regular basis, toxins can build up in the system. This common problem can often be corrected with diet, lifestyle changes, and natural remedies. However, if constipation continues, see your physician or a natural health practitioner to evaluate and treat the underlying problem. Another consideration might be to try a colonic irrigation. These are performed by certified practitioners and can help to rid the body of sludge buildup in the colon.

It is unfortunate that many people are told that having a bowel movement a few times per week is normal for them. This may true in that this person moves their bowels this number of times per week, but it is far from optimal for health concerns. If you were to visit tribesmen in the Amazon you would note that they have a bowel movement approximately thirty minutes after each and every meal. This is optimal!

I have a family member that was in this very predicament. After she had a series of colonic irrigations she began to move her bowels once or twice per day and has felt much better because of this.

Diarrhea is generally caused by foods that have an overabundance of harmful bacteria, water that has been contaminated with harmful organisms, allergies to foods, or stress.

Any of these factors can stimulate increased peristaltic activity. When food moves through the digestive tract too rapidly, there is less ability to digest and assimilate what you eat. This can also be the digestive tract's attempt to rid the body of toxins or microbes. In some cases, diarrhea is the body's intelligence at work. Exposure to harmful microorganisms tends to be more frequent than most of us realize, for example, from food when you eat out, or from drinking water containing microscopic germs, such as Cryptosporidium.

If diarrhea is the body's attempt to rid itself of harmful organisms, we should allow it to do just that! Stopping diarrhea in this type of situation is foolish. Medicines that slow down intestinal activity are commonly used for acute and chronic diarrhea. Probiotics often help calm diarrhea because the healthy bacteria counters infections. Other natural remedies that can help clear problem microbes include grapefruit seed extract, garlic, ginger, plant tannins, and oil of oregano capsules.

If diarrhea persists, get checked out for parasites and pathogenic bacteria. If the problem is ongoing or chronic, consider asking for antibody testing. This approach is currently the state-of-the-art in testing for GI problems, using a simple blood test, or a saliva testing. Antibodies are tiny proteins in the blood that show if your body has "fought off" a particular germ. For example, antibody testing is widely used to indicate if someone has had the measles or had an infection with H. pylori bacteria. Your doctor can request any of a number of antibody tests that include: Microflora competence, which checks for yeast and several different types of bacteria, and or IgA testing for parasites, which checks for twelve different kinds of parasites, including giardia and amoebas.

Gas and bloating is the result of eating too fast, combining foods that do not agree with your system, allergies, intestinal yeast overgrowth, fermentation of food (such as meat that takes up to forty eight hours to digest), or those harmful microorganisms we've discussed earlier. When food is not digested properly, it can easily ferment in the digestive tract and lead to nausea, indigestion, gas, and bloating. Toxins produced by harmful microorganisms get absorbed into the bloodstream and affect energy levels, one's mood, and brain function.

Some of the solutions for gas and bloating include watching your eating habits, chewing thoroughly and relaxing while you eat. You should avoid drinking liquids with meals or right before eating unless you are trying to lose weight. Liquid dilutes your digestive acids and enzymes. When you are attempting to lose some unwanted pounds you should drink a large glass of water fifteen to thirty minutes prior to eating a meal. This will suppress your appetite and give you the feeling of being full.

If symptoms persist for weeks, seek the help of a physician and let him/her evaluate your lifestyle to find the source of your problem. Your physician should also check for yeast, parasites, and other harmful microorganisms. There are many helpful natural remedies that may include probiotics, grapefruit seed extract, peppermint tea, tumeric powder in capsules, and fennel or anise seeds. I have found activated charcoal capsules to be very effective in treating gas and bloating and they are extremely inexpensive.

Food sensitivities can cause poor digestion or allergy-like digestive reactions. Any of the above problems such as heartburn, as well as problems like headaches, congested sinuses, achy joints, or fatigue can cause these symptoms. Pay attention to what you are eating and how you feel after you eat it. A reaction to a certain food can be almost instant in some cases, or it may take hours to develop. If food sensitivity is a major issue for you, try keeping a food diary to track how you interact with foods. You may want to try eating only one food at a meal or even one food a day to determine what is triggering your response. The most typical causes of food reactions are the sensitive seven: cow's milk, wheat, sugar, corn, eggs, peanuts, and soy products.

Avoiding any problematic foods will obviously alleviate the problem. Since food reactions are also associated with intestinal bugs or incomplete digestion, finding the basic cause of your sensitivity may take some systematic work with your health care practitioner. Supplements that can help to reduce food reactions are Vitamin C, quercetin, glutamine, bicarbonate, hydrochloric acid, charcoal capsules, and aloe vera juice (with lemon).

There are a variety of food allergy tests, also referred to as food sensitivity testing (both food antibody assessment and cell reaction tests). A variety of labs offer these tests, but not all doctors use them. Find a practitioner in your area who is familiar with food sensitivity problems.

Let's take a look at some of the digestive supplements that may help with your problem. We all need the natural hydrochloric acid produced in our stomach to help digest proteins and fats. Due to chronic stress and poor diets, many people actually do not have enough stomach acid, and this is common in the elderly. Often we reach for an antacid to alleviate stomach distress, when in fact we are lacking digestive acids to properly digest our food.

If you feel that you are not digesting efficiently, try a product called betaine hydrochloride with pepsin (a time-released protein digestant), available at health food stores. These capsule(s) are taken after you begin eating, so the supplement mixes in with your food, which is especially helpful for digesting meals rich in protein or fats. Try one capsule for the first couple of meals; if that feels okay, you can try two and gradually increase to three or four capsules. If you have any sensation of burning or acid indigestion, stop the supplement. You can try cutting back to a more comfortable level again in a day or two. Monitor your digestion to see if it has improved. Some people who have allergies, food reactions, or even eczema benefit from taking additional hydrochloric acid. In addition, take time to eat, chew your food well, and avoid stress. These are the basics to promote good digestion.

Lack of sufficient pancreatic enzymes is another common cause of incomplete digestion, resulting from chronic stress, overeating, poor food choices, or possibly infection. Of particular value are specially coated enzymes that survive the stomach's acid environment (called "enteric coated"). Digestive enzymes come in bottles of powdered capsules and chewable tablets. There are different qualities and combinations; some are even vegetarian formulas. I recommend taking one to two or three capsules after you eat to add enzymes to the food once it has begun to be digested. Chewing well and taking time to eat your food is the best way to get your digestive tract to work the way it should. Making the right food choices for your body is also helpful.

Bicarbonate is an over-the-counter remedy and is useful when the goal is to minimize excess stomach acid or to control acid or allergic type reactions. Most people with poor digestion need more stomach acid, rather than less. During detox programs, when your body is clearing acid wastes, bicarbonate can be useful. This can be used as regular baking soda, or buffered Vitamin C formulas with calcium and other alkaline minerals, or the many typical antacids available in the stores. Antacids could contain aluminum or other harmful chemicals, and should be used as a last resort.

If you have any burning sensation in your belly take as directed, or use one-half to one teaspoon of baking soda after or between meals. Good intestinal bacteria, called probiotics, help us digest our food, and they are important in our ability to resist illness. Taking probiotics when indicated, or with digestive upset (Aloe Vera juice or gel may also help), or following use of antibiotics, or when traveling to protect against harmful microorganisms. Beware when you're traveling, because you still want to be sure to take every precaution against harmful microorganisms--probiotics are not an automatic protection. Take them after antibiotics, which can alter GI flora, using probiotics in concentrated powder or liquid form. Beneficial bacteria include lactobacillus acidophilus, bifidobacteria, lactobacillus bulgaricus, and sacchromyces boulardii. I usually recommend taking your probiotics on an empty stomach, or if that is not possible, take them a minimum of twenty minutes before or after your meals or first thing in the morning and right before bed. One or two capsules or between a quarter and half-teaspoon is typical or follow the directions on the bottle.

Yogurt appears to provide a source of healthy flora. We know that in societies where people (the Eastern Europeans for example) eat yogurt routinely, they have a history of living exceptionally long and healthy lives. So consider yogurt as a possible source of flora, especially fresh, homemade yogurt or a reliable brand. Check the label for the type and quantity of organisms and to see if there is added sugar. Certain brands may agree with you better than others. Some people, for example, find excellent results with brands that are also high in bifidobacteria. Be sure to read labels and track your responses. Remember that food tolerances are always very individual responses.

Beware of food sensitivities. The first consideration with yogurt is to be sure you don't have a dairy allergy or sensitivity. Some people with dairy allergies can still tolerate yogurt every few days. People who can't handle cow's milk yogurt may want to try goat's milk yogurt, or even soy acidophilus.

Lactobacillus acidophilus is the culture found in most yogurts. When ulcerative colitis was treated with eight different strains of acidophilus and bifidobacteria, twelve of fifteen patients experienced long-term remission in a small study by the University of Bologna.

Lactobacillus DDS is one of the more studied acidophilus strains and is the DDS strain which is available nationwide in health food stores. It has been documented in research to survive storage in dry form in the capsule on the shelf, and to produce viable cultures in the gastrointestinal tract, and to boost GI immunity. (Look for products that say DDS strain.)

In a study of children with recurrent abdominal pain, they were given a form of lactobacilli plantarum. Of these, sixty percent experienced a decrease in pain over the four-week period, in a study by the University of Nebraska.

Irritable bowel syndrome treated with L. plantarum found rates of improvement of sixty seven to ninety percent, in a study conducted in a Polish hospital. Patients who used drug therapy improved by thirty percent, and those who took the placebo (with no medication or flora) showed no improvement.

Sacchromyces Boulardii is another frequently recommended supplement, which is naturally occurring in yeast, and a close relative of baker's yeast. It stimulates the production of secretory IgA (protective antibodies in the lining of the digestive tract). There have been a number of studies indicating that this yeast in supplement form can decrease the course of GI illness.

Traveler's diarrhea was effectively treated with S. boulardiiin in a group of ninety five German patients. Of these, sixty seven percent had failed to respond to previous anti-diarrhea or antibiotic drugs.

Colitis associated with Clostridium difficile responded well to the use of S. boulardii, which was used in conjunction with the antibiotics vancomycin and metronidazole in a study by the University of West Virginia.

S. Boulardii was found to prevent diarrhea in critically ill tube-fed patients in a French study.

Soil-based bacteria, also known as homeostatic soil organisms, are gaining attention as viable GI flora. HSOs are an addition to the usual probiotic agents such as lactobacillus and bifidobacteria. Like other forms of flora, they are exceptionally helpful to some patients and moderately helpful to others. The theory is when most people lived on farms they took in these natural substances as part of their food.

An overgrowth of yeast (candida) and bacteria can be checked through the CDSA, and presence of these organisms (and parasites) can also be discovered by antibody testing, which is available through health practitioners.

Many patients comment that the choice of treatments and remedies is overwhelming. What to do? How do you know if you need more acid or less? Which vitamins? Which herbs? Everything you do requires some careful experimentation. Solutions develop out of your experience and your observation of the results. Your awareness is the key.

Try some of these simple remedies first. If they haven't worked in a few weeks, your doctor or natural medicine practitioner can also perform some simple testing to focus in on the cause of the problem.

Preventing & Treating Digestive Problems in a Nutshell

- Eat in a relaxed way in a pleasant setting, and take your time.
- Chew your food until it is liquid.

- If you are under emotional pressure or in a hurry, eat or drink simple foods such as fresh juice, a fruit, yogurt, a few nuts or seeds, or a protein bar.
- Keep up your exercise regimen. Walking and yoga are both particularly good for digestion.
- Drink plenty of fresh water (approximately sixty four to eighty ounces), but not with meals unless you're on a weight-loss diet trying to lower food intake.
- Minimize ice cold drinks and consume more soothing warm drinks such as hot lemon water or herb teas.
- Get plenty of fiber in your diet, whether from vegetables, fruits, bran or psyllium, and an adequate amount of whole grains and fresh sprouts.
- Remove food allergens from your diet. Learn which foods cause reactions and affect how you feel.
- Minimize toxins and irritants; eat organic foods whenever possible, and eat simply. People who have digestive disorders should avoid additives, such as fluoride (often added to toothpaste), and carageenan (found in cottage cheese and other foods), both of which can act as irritants.
- If you have chronic indigestion, try supplementing your meals with enzymes and/or hydrochloric acid. If that doesn't help, ask your doctor to test you for these factors. Then, supplement as needed with enzymes (to aid digestion), bicarbonate soda (for excess acid), or betaine hydrochloride capsules (for deficient stomach acid).
- Learn your best personal remedies for digestive upsets. You can learn to minimize constipation and diarrhea by using foods, herbs, and nutrients that help to prevent these common ailments and cope with them when they do occur.
- Occasional indigestion, heartburn, bloating after you eat, and flatulence are normal, or at least quite common, and they can be remedied. But, if you have ongoing symptoms of digestive upset, get tested to see if you have food allergies, low or high stomach acid, yeast overgrowth, or bad microorganisms.

- Support and repair the digestive tract with the right nutrients, such as glutamine and other vitamins and minerals.
- Eat a low allergenic diet, find the best foods that feel right to you, and chew your food well.[40]

---

[40] http://www.elsonhaas.com/articles/article_11.html, Causes & Remedies for Common Digestive Problems, Elson Haas, MD, 11/27/06.

Conclusion

I will never be an old man. To me, old age is always 15 years older than I am.
Francis Bacon

One of the goals of this book, and a life's mission of mine, is to help people understand that they are ultimately responsible for their own health, and that the choices they make on a daily basis will affect their health in the future. Your health level is not something that just happens. It is up to each and every individual to make the best out of their circumstance in life by gaining knowledge and understanding and putting these things into action.

I've been told that I am a health fanatic. I hope I am because a fanatic is someone who is doing a little more than most people want to do. Why do I do the things I've outlined in this book? The answer is because I believe whole heartedly in what I've written. If you ask me how I will be working on my health and fitness in another decade, I would have to say I am not sure, because I too am on a journey and hopefully I will acquire some new techniques and tools to use on my personal journey.

You can look and feel great after fifty, but it does take some effort on your part. There is no magic bullet that will transform you into the body of a healthy twenty year old. Our nation is in the midst of a health care crisis because we want everything fast and easy. Just drive up to the fast food window and tell the doctor that you want to alleviate certain symptoms; never mind taking care of the problem. It just doesn't work that way!

Everyone likes a money back guarantee, so here it is: I can guarantee if you were to incorporate some, or all of the concepts I've given in this book, you will look and feel better than you do now. After all, isn't that what we are all looking to do when we purchase a book like this one?

257

Some of the concepts given in this book require more effort than others, but each has merit worthy of the effort. When I read a book about health and or fitness, I generally find one or more concepts that I try, and if they show promise I continue to do them. If you are the type of person who has a difficult time with self discipline then pick one concept from this book and give it a try for a month. Perhaps it will be drinking more pure water every day, or maybe you will begin to walk on a regular basis. Whichever one you try give it a month and you will be pleasantly surprised on the outcome.

The next month continue to do the thing you started last month, and now add one more health producing item to your lifestyle. If you did this for a year you would eventually have a healthy lifestyle that will give you great rewards for your efforts.

The people that I chose to do bios on are, in my opinion, healthy and fit. They are not perfect specimens of the human body, and neither am I for that matter, but they are a work in progress. They too are on a journey. Some of these people may have some bad habits, just as you or I probably have, but they are working with the knowledge and ability they have and are benefitting from it. We can all improve our current levels of health and fitness. All we have to do is take that first step, and then the second step and then the third step, and you will find that with each step you take in the right direction it starts to become a pleasant walk.

You can do it! The reason I can say that with such conviction is because I am a firm believer that if one person can do it, then you and I can do it as well. Perhaps you will be the next person that someone will write about when you are one hundred and twenty years young!

You have been given some good sound advice outlined in this book. Now it is up to you, the reader, to take action on what you now know!

Grow old with me! The best is yet to be.
Robert Browning

258

Recommended Reading and Reference Material

1. "Prescriptions for Nutritional Healing" by Phyllis A. Balch, CNC & James F. Balch, MD
2. "Dr. John Lee's Hormone Balance Made Simple"
3. "Illustrated Yoga" by Moran
4. "Super Foods" by Steven Pratt, MD & Kathy Matthews
5. "The Arthritis Cure" by Theodosakis, Adderly & Fox
6. "Dr. Jensen's Guide to Better Bowel Care"
7. "The Anti-Aging Zone" by Barry Sears, PhD

If you would like to contact Dr. Fisher for a personal consultation online go to: www.naturopathicdoctorsoffice.com

Index

.